easy to ma

Low GI

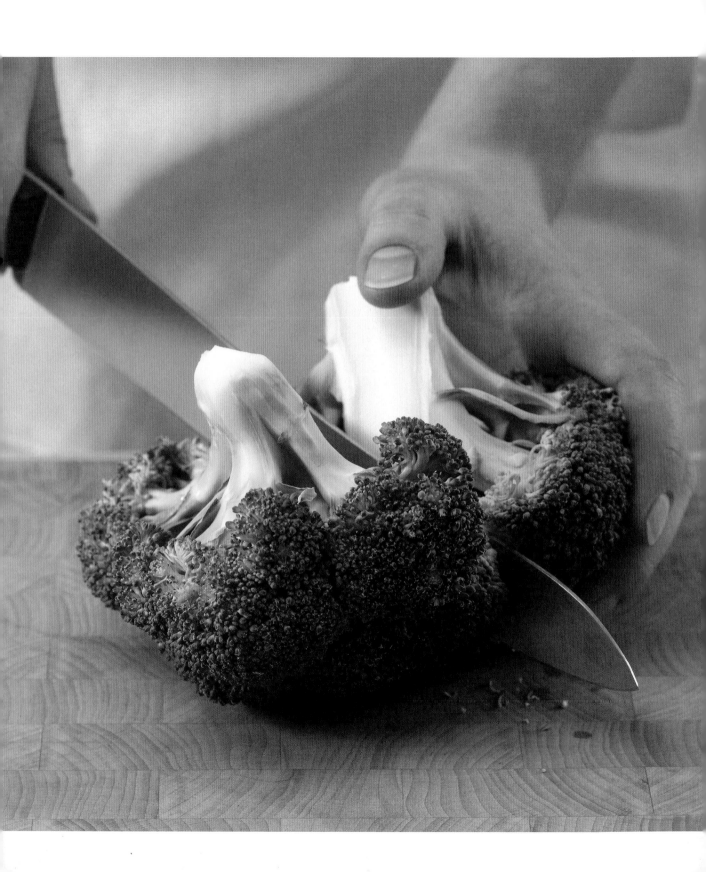

Good Housekeeping

easy to make!
Low GI

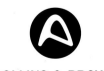

COLLINS & BROWN

First published in Great Britain in 2008
by Collins & Brown
10 Southcombe Street
London W14 0RA

An imprint of Anova Books Company Ltd

The Good Housekeeping website is
www.goodhousekeeping.co.uk

10 9 8 7 6 5 4 3 2

ISBN 978-1-84340-466-8

A catalogue record for this book is available from the British
Library.

Reproduction by Dot Gradations Ltd
Printed and bound by SNP Leefung, China

Keep updated. Email food@anovabooks.com

This book can be ordered direct from the publisher. Contact the
marketing department, but try your bookshop first.

www.anovabooks.com

NOTES

- Both metric and imperial measures are given for the recipes. Follow either set of measures, not a mixture of both, as they are not interchangeable.
- All spoon measures are level.
  1 tsp = 5ml spoon; 1 tbsp = 15ml spoon.
- Ovens and grills must be preheated to the specified temperature.
- Use sea salt and freshly ground black pepper unless otherwise suggested.
- Fresh herbs should be used unless dried herbs are specified in a recipe.
- Medium eggs should be used except where otherwise specified. Free-range eggs are recommended.
- Note that certain recipes, including mayonnaise, lemon curd and some cold desserts, contain raw or lightly cooked eggs. The young, elderly, pregnant women and anyone with an immune-deficiency disease should avoid these, because of the slight risk of salmonella.
- Calorie, fat and carbohydrate counts per serving are provided for the recipes.

Picture Credits
Photographers: Steve Baxter (page 110); Linda Burgess (page 124); Nicki Dowey (pages 34, 37, 39, 40, 41, 48, 49, 51, 53, 55, 56, 58, 60, 62, 64, 65, 71, 72, 75, 76, 79, 81, 82, 84, 85, 86, 87, 89, 90, 94, 95, 97, 99, 101, 102, 105, 111, 112, 115, 118, 121, 122 and126); Will Heap (pages 35, 36, 46, 67, 74, 77, 80, 98, 100, 107, 116, 119 and 125); Craig Robertson (all Basics photography); Lucinda Symons (pages 32, 33, 38, 44, 45, 50, 54, 59, 61, 70, 91 and 104)
Stylist: Helen Trent
Home Economists: Emma Jane Frost and Teresa Goldfinch

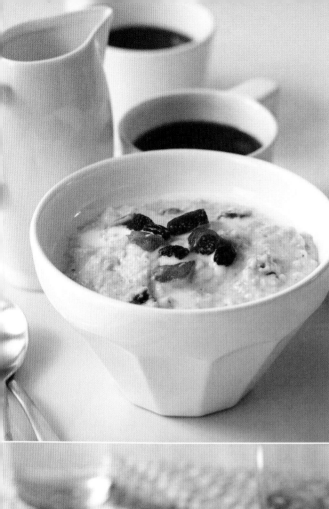

Contents

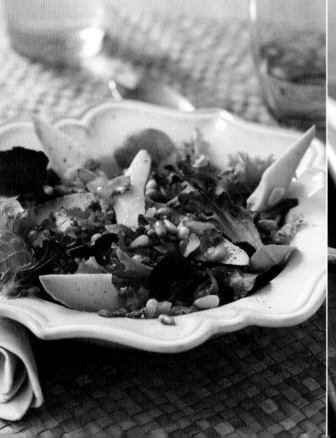

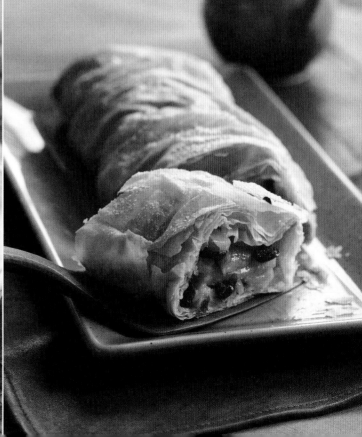

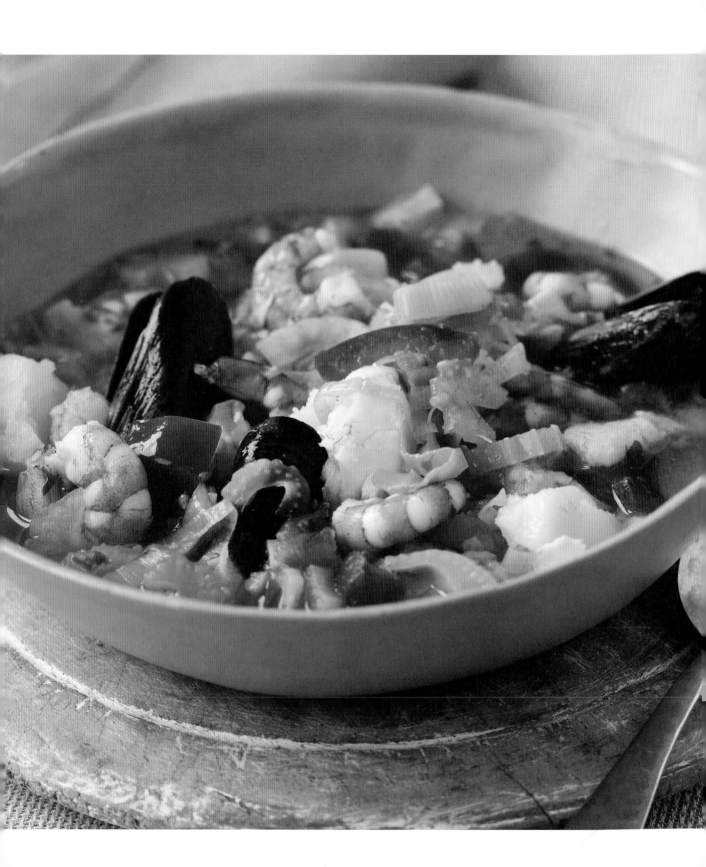

Foreword

The glycaemic index (GI) diet is not a weight-loss fad, but a common-sense approach to healthy eating – for life. The glycaemic index was developed to help diabetics keep their blood sugar levels steady: it is a measure of how quickly foods are broken down by the body to provide energy. It soon became clear that everyone, not just diabetics, could benefit from eating food that releases energy slowly. Choosing low-GI food can help you lose weight because you will feel fuller for longer, with fewer hunger pangs, mood swings and energy dips. But even if you don't need to lose weight, the glycaemic index is vitally important: eating low-GI foods can stabilise the body's production of insulin, which can help you to avoid developing insulin resistance (sometimes called Syndrome X), potentially leading to life-threatening conditions such as diabetes, strokes and heart attacks. The good news is that it's very easy to switch to a low-GI lifestyle, as this book shows. Low GI includes a clear, concise guide to the glycaemic index, with lists of low-, medium- and high-GI foods, tips on reducing the GI of the food you eat and techniques to make preparing low-GI food as quick and easy as possible. The recipes take you through the day, from breakfast to light lunches, quick suppers and food for entertaining friends, with a tempting selection of treats for the sweet-toothed.

We've gathered together 101 ideas for feeding your family the low-GI way. All the recipes have been triple tested in the Good Housekeeping kitchens to make sure they work every time.

Emma

Emma Marsden
Cookery Editor
Good Housekeeping

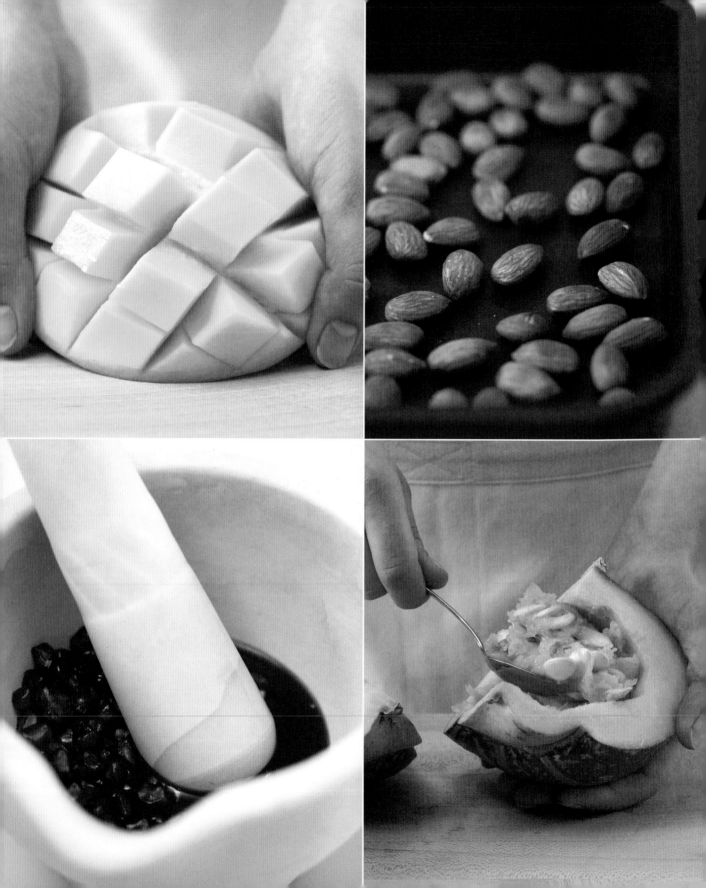

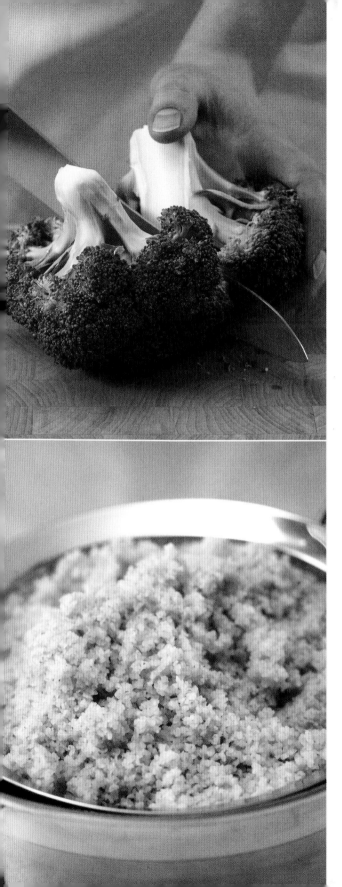

0

The Basics

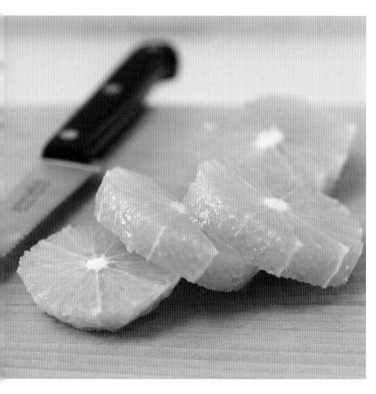

What are GI foods?

GI foods are carbohydrate foods, and any food that contains carbohydrate, in the form of starch, sugar or fibre, will have a GI ranking. Pure glucose produces the greatest rise in blood sugar levels. Because of this it has been given a GI rating of 100 and is used as a standard by which other foods are ranked. All other foods are ranked from 0–100. See the table on page 12.

Low GI: 0–55
Medium GI: 55–70
High GI: 70–100

Note: Although the rankings are useful, because different foods affect GI levels, it is the overall balance of the foods you eat in a day that counts, not just individual GI values.

What's the difference between high- and low-GI foods?

High-GI foods break down quickly in the body, causing a rapid release of glucose (blood sugar) into your bloodstream. Foods high in processed starch, such as white bread, highly refined breakfast cereals and pastries, are all high-GI foods. Low-GI foods, by contrast, such as pulses, wholegrain foods and most fruit and vegetables, break down slowly, causing a steady and sustained release of glucose into the bloodstream.

Why are high-GI foods bad for you?

Releasing high amounts of glucose into your bloodstream causes your body to go into red alert – too much is harmful – and to produce high levels of insulin (which regulates glucose and enables excess to be stored as fat). The net effect is the familiar yo-yo of 'sugar highs' followed by 'sugar lows' (energy dips), sugar cravings, mood swings and general fatigue. In time, insulin resistance, diabetes and other severe illnesses can develop. It's also thought that, for various reasons, high-GI foods are counterproductive and actually stimulate the appetite, rather than curb it, and are a significant factor in weight gain.

What is GI?

GI stands for Glycaemic Index, and is a measure of how slowly or quickly carbohydrates in the food you eat break down to glucose in your body. It is glucose – the simplest form of sugar – that your body and brain use as fuel, both in every living process and to provide you with energy. Whether you have too much, too little or a steady flow of glucose in your bloodstream is fundamental to your overall health, and is the key to weight control, how you feel emotionally, and whether you feel tired or full of energy.

Why are low-GI foods good for you?

Low-GI foods avoid all the pitfalls of high-GI foods. In addition, because often they are more nutritious, they are good value foods. Choosing them is the easy way to ensure your diet is a healthy one. Research also suggests low-GI eating results in a higher level of good HDL cholesterol, which helps to protect against heart disease.

How do I know which foods are low-GI or high-GI?

GI values have been worked out for most foods containing carbohydrates, and you can buy books that contain only this information. Some manufactured foods in supermarkets also have GI values printed on their packaging. However, for practical purposes, all you need to know is which foods are high-GI foods and which are low. The chart on page 12 lists low-, medium- and high-GI foods to help you plan your dishes and menus.

What about proteins and fats?

Fats, oils and protein foods (meat, poultry, fish and eggs) do not contain carbohydrates, and therefore have no GI values. However, this does not mean that you can eat as much of them as you like. The usual healthy eating rules apply. All, especially fats, are energy-dense foods, and should be eaten in moderation, while your intake of saturated and processed (hydrogenated) fats should be kept to a minimum.
Dairy products that contain lactose (milk, yogurt and some cheeses) have low-GI ratings.
Protein and fats slow down digestion of carbohydrates, and lower its GI. This is why, for example, although they are energy-dense foods, nuts and seeds are low GI.

What about fibre?

The presence of soluble fibre in food – for example, in oats, beans, and in fruits such as apples and pears – lowers GI. This is one of the reasons why dried beans and pulses are star low-GI foods.

What else affects GI?

GI is a measure of the rate at which carbohydrates are digested. The following factors affect this rate, and therefore the GI value of the food:

- Cooking, mashing and processing
- Acidity
- The amount of protein and fat present
- The amount of carbohydrate and fibre present

What about low-GI weight-reducing diets?

Low-GI weight-reducing diets, combined with exercise, have been shown to be very effective, and are thought to be one of the best ways to maintain your weight safely. They usually also incorporate a low-fat regime.

Low-GI foods:

0–55 GI

All green vegetables, onions and leeks

All salad vegetables, and herbs

Sprouted seeds and bean sprouts

Carrots, artichokes, celeriac

Avocado

Sweet potatoes, yams

Apples, pears, stone fruits – nectarines, plums, gages, peaches and apricots – and soft fruit such as strawberries, blueberries and other berries

Citrus fruits

Fruit and vegetable juices

Dried apples, pears, apricots, mango, prunes

Durum wheat pasta – all kinds

Egg pasta and noodles

Glass and cellophane noodles (made from pea and bean flour)

Grain breads containing whole seeds and nuts; pumpernickel bread

Stoneground wholewheat and rye breads

Stoneground oats, rolled oats

Nuts and seeds

All dried beans and pulses

Canned beans; sugar-reduced baked beans

Brown, red and wild rice

Bulgur wheat, buckwheat, quinoa, amaranth, pearl barley

Breakfast cereals and mueslis containing whole (not flaked) grains; sugar-free muesli, All Bran

Meat, poultry, eggs and fish

Dairy products

Fats and oils

Plain milk and plain dark chocolate

Medium-GI foods:

55–70 GI

Basmati rice

Couscous

Polenta

Rice noodles

Beetroot, swede, winter squashes (pumpkins)

Sweetcorn

Tropical fruits*: banana, kiwi fruit, mango, papaya/paw-paw, pineapple

Cherries, grapes

Fresh dates

Dried cranberries, figs, raisins, sultanas

Sugar

Honey

Maple syrup

Most jams and preserves

Most chocolates

* Amber fruits have GI values in the mid-to-high 50s. All are valuable sources of nutrients, so do not let their GI ranking deter you from eating them.

High-GI foods:

70–100 GI

Processed breakfast cereals such as cornflakes, Rice Crispies, puffed grain cereals, crunchies, millet flakes, instant porridge oats; some mueslis

Processed white and brown breads, white flour

Savoury and sweet pastries

Most cakes and biscuits; croissants, crumpets

Processed savoury and sweet snacks

Crispbreads, crackers, rice cakes and popcorn

Canned soft and sports drinks

Risotto, pudding, sticky and quick-cook long-grain rice varieties

Gluten-free pasta and some noodles

Potatoes in all forms: for example, mashed, roast

Broad beans

Cooked parsnips

Watermelon

Dried dates

Liquorice

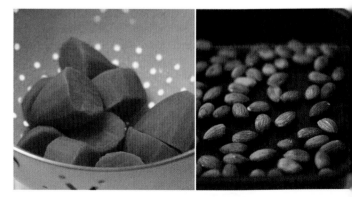

Benefits of a low-GI lifestyle

Ensures you eat plenty of fresh, wholesome, healthy unprocessed foods.
Keeps you feeling satisfied for longer, so avoids hunger pangs.
Controls appetite by ensuring stable reduced levels of blood sugar and insulin.
Banishes energy dips and mood swings.
Maximises burning of fat by reducing blood sugar levels.
Helps protect against diabetes and heart disease.
Ensures steady weight loss.
Results in a slimmer, more energised, healthier, happier you.

In the kitchen

Switching to a low-GI lifestyle requires no radical changes to your diet or daily eating pattern – indeed, that is part of its attraction. Nor does it mean only eating low-GI foods. It simply means altering the balance away from high-GI foods to low-GI foods, which take longer to digest and thus make you feel fuller for longer, and getting into the habit, whenever possible, of serving low-GI foods at every meal. The good news is that making some very simple changes can make a huge difference. For example, just eating one low-GI food at every meal will mean glucose and insulin levels stay lower all day.

Top Tips

The golden rule is that the more starch has been processed or cooked, the higher its GI is likely to be.
Reduce highly processed foods, such as white bread products, breakfast cereals and pastries, sugary foods, confectionery, cakes, biscuits and canned soft and sports drinks as much as you can.
Substitute lower-GI equivalents of high-GI staples – bread, breakfast cereals, rice.
When you eat high-GI foods, eat them in smaller portions.
Remember to always cook pasta al dente, until just tender but still firm to the bite; overcooking increases its GI value.
Combine high-GI with low-GI foods to slow down the rate at which high-GI foods are broken down, reducing their effects.
Include lean protein/fresh vegetables/fresh fruit/salads/pulses/nuts and seeds, whichever is appropriate when you eat, so that you will always be eating low-GI foods at every meal.
Acidity lowers the rate of digestion of high-GI foods – for example, using lemon or lime juice or natural yogurt, eating half a grapefruit for breakfast, using a vinaigrette/balsamic dressing for salads.
Choose fresh fruit or fruit canned in natural juice instead of in syrup.

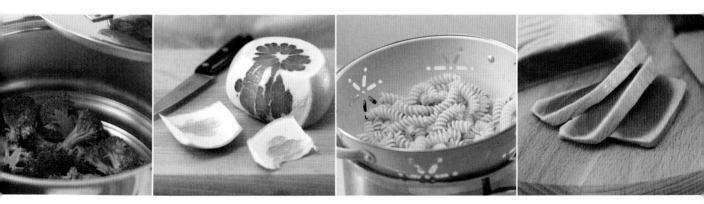

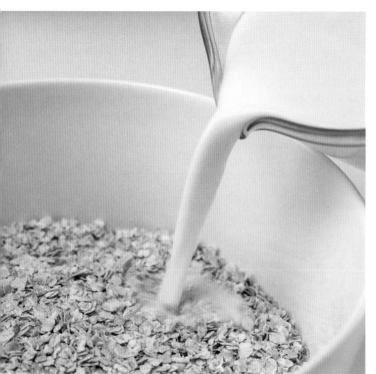

Get smart: know your carbs

The secret to adapting to a low-GI eating plan is to substitute high-GI carbs for better low/medium-GI carbs, most of the time.

Bread

✗ White and brown processed breads in all forms have the highest GI ratings.
✓ Wholegrain, Granary, pumpernickel and seed breads, stoneground wholewheat and rye breads, sourdough breads.

Breakfast cereals

✗ Processed breakfast cereals such as Shredded Wheat, Rice Crispies, instant porridge oats, puffed grain cereals, cornflakes and those high in added sugar or honey such as crunchies and cereal bars.
✓ Porridge made with traditional rolled oats or stoneground oatmeal; sugar-free/low-sugar mueslis, All Bran.

Pasta

✗ As long as you eat smaller than normal portions and do not overcook it, pasta is generally OK. Rice noodles are medium-high GI and gluten-free pasta (which is often made from corn) is high GI.
✓ All kinds of durum wheat pasta; fresh pasta made with eggs; cellophane and glass noodles (which are made from pea and bean flours).

Rice

✗ Most varieties of white long-grain rice, including processed American long-grain, jasmine rice, and all short round varieties such as pudding, risotto and sticky glutinous rice.
✓ White and brown basmati, brown, red and wild rice.

Potatoes

✗ All potatoes: boiled, mashed, fried, instant, and so on.
✓ Boiled new potatoes (these are still high-GI, but are significantly lower than maincrop potatoes); sweet potatoes and yams.

Sugar

Though it's sensible to use as little sugar as possible, the only form of sugar that is high GI is glucose. Table sugar (sucrose) and honey are medium GI; the sugar found in fresh fruit (fructose) is low GI. You can now buy low-GI fruit sugar to replace table sugar in tea and coffee and in baking. This is expensive, but you need one-third less. When baking with fruit sugar, reduce the cooking temperature by 25°C.

Chocolate

Generally, chocolates and bars tend to have medium-GI values. Because of their added sugar and fat, however, they are still indulgence foods. Dark plain chocolate, with a minimum of 70% cocoa solids, is low GI. Milk chocolate is also low GI, but is less healthy than dark chocolate because it contains more fat and sugar.

Dried fruits

These are low to medium GI. The one exception is dates, which are extremely high GI and have a GI value of 100.

Low-GI snacks

Everyone needs to snack sometimes. Resist the temptation to reach for the biscuits or processed snacks, and tuck into these healthy low-GI snacks instead.

Fresh fruit, nuts and seeds are ideal low-GI foods. Make sure you take some of each with you whenever you go out, or travel.

Dried apricots and prunes are delicious nutrient-packed low-GI snacks, and are the perfect handy snack instead of sweets.

Keep a dip and crudités in the fridge for emergency snacking. Good dips are mashed avocado (guacamole) and hummus. Mayonnaise blended with a little mustard and natural yogurt is excellent also.

An avocado is a light meal in itself, highly nutritious – a good source of EFAs (essential fatty acids) and vitamin E – and will keep hunger pangs at bay. Spoon a little extra virgin olive oil or your favourite health oil into the cavity and enjoy.

A couple of squares of dark plain chocolate (70% cocoa solids) is a permissible treat, and better than a sugary snack.

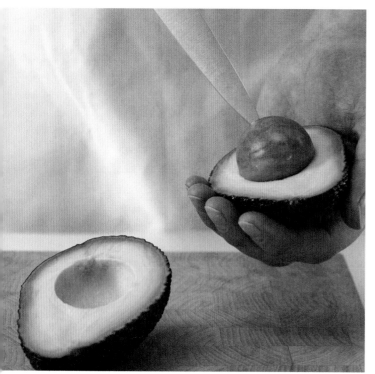

Healthy living

A low-GI diet ensures you eat plenty of unrefined, good carbohydrates, and will play a significant part in keeping you healthy and energised. Incorporating low-GI eating into a healthy lifestyle, by following these ten simple steps, will set you up for life and ensure you achieve maximum health and vitality.

Ten easy steps to health

1. Water

Water is the elixir of life, and is nature's prime detoxifier.
- Aim to drink at least 1 litre (1³/₄ pints) per day, preferably 1–2 litres (1³/₄–3¹/₂ pints).
- Start the day with a glass of hot water and lemon.
- Have a small bottle or a large glass of mineral or filtered water by your side always, and sip regularly.
- Drinking water at room temperature is easier on the digestion than ice-cold water.
- Bored with plain water? Flavour your water with a slice of lemon, lime or some peeled and chopped fresh ginger.

2. Superfoods

For tiptop nutrition and long-term health, incorporate these foods into your regular eating plan:

Avocado
Broccoli
Carrots
Cabbage
Garlic
Ripe tomatoes
Sprouted seeds: for example, alfalfa
Watercress
Winter squash (dense orange-fleshed varieties such as butternut)
Apples
Apricots
Bananas
Berries
Kiwi fruit
Lemons
Pineapple
Live, natural yogurt
Miso
Oats
Sea vegetables (seaweed): for example, nori strips

3. Good fats and oils

Fats are essential to all life processes, including the production of cholesterol, which is vital for nerve communication and an essential component of the brain, nerve fibres and sex hormones. For this reason, a low-fat diet is not a good idea for long-term health. The trick is to substitute bad (processed, hydrogenated and highly saturated) fats for omega-rich good fats and oils, found in oily fish, nuts and seeds, and to eat small amounts of other natural fats such as olive oil and butter.

- Eat 1–2 tbsp extra virgin (cold pressed) oils every day. Olive oil, hemp, linseed and blends of omega oils are especially good. Do not heat. Use them to drizzle over salads, vegetables and fish, and in dips.

4. Vegetables, salads and fruit

Vegetables, salads and fruit are star performers in all healthy eating plans, including low-GI ones. Not only do they contain a storehouse of vitamins and minerals, they also help to keep the body at its optimum pH, which is slightly alkaline.

5. Eat regularly

Skipping meals leads to energy dips, stresses your system and is a sure-fire way to put on weight. Eating regularly keeps your body's physical and mental energy levels steady, avoiding hunger pangs and the need to snack.

- Never skip breakfast – it's the most important meal of the day to set you up and it also sustains your energy levels through until lunchtime.
- Eat slowly, and take your time – it takes 20 minutes for your body to register it is full and satiated.

6. Variety

Enjoy as wide a variety of foods as possible. This way you will ensure your diet contains all the health-giving micronutrients it needs for optimum health. It also helps to avoid developing intolerances to particular foods.

7. Exercise

Regular exercise is vital, and is a crucial ingredient in all low-GI weight-reducing diets. It energises you, raises your metabolic rate, helps to maintain your correct weight, is a de-stressor, releases feel-good hormones, and helps you sleep better.

8. Stress less

Stress is a major modern disease and comes in all shapes and sizes, be it pressure at work, from noise and traffic, or the constant barrage of environmental and electronic pollution. The body reacts to stress by going into red alert and your immune system is compromised. Learning to deal with stress, and removing stress from your life wherever you can, is essential for your health.

- Build some form of relaxation into your daily life.
- Learn simple deep breathing techniques.
- Reduce the hours you watch TV or work/play on the computer. Listen to soothing music instead.

9. Sleep

Sleep is Nature's happy pill, the ultimate physical and mental reviver, and the secret to staying young. Take care of your sleep and your body and your immune system will take care of you. Make getting enough sleep a top priority.

- Make your bedroom a peaceful haven.
- Avoid drinking coffee or too much alcohol in the evening.
- Wind down before you go to bed.

10. Positive outlook

How you feel has a critical impact on your health and overall wellbeing. Cultivate an optimistic outlook and do something that makes you happy every day. Laughter is great medicine, and is completely free.

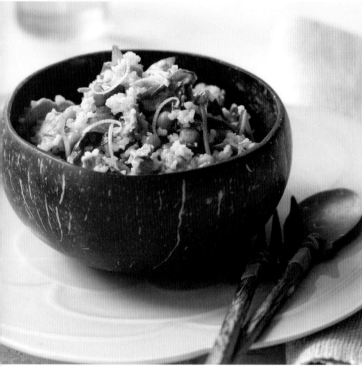

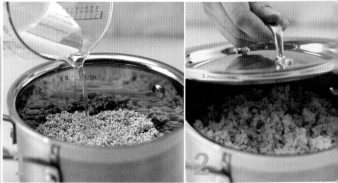

Quinoa

This nutritious South American grain makes a great alternative to rice.

1 Put the quinoa in a bowl of cold water. Mix well, soak for 2 minutes, then drain. Put in a pan with twice its volume of water. Bring to the boil.

2 Simmer for 20 minutes. Remove from the heat, cover and leave to stand for 10 minutes.

Using grains

Grains such as wheat, barley and quinoa are the edible seeds of different grasses. Many of these grains are available in a variety of forms; as side dishes they make good low-GI alternatives to rice and potatoes.

Pearl barley

Barley comes in several forms, so you should check which type you have bought.

Pearl barley has had its outer husk removed, and needs no soaking. Rinse the barley in cold water, then put it in a pan with twice its volume of water. Bring to the boil. Turn down the heat and simmer until tender, 25–30 minutes.

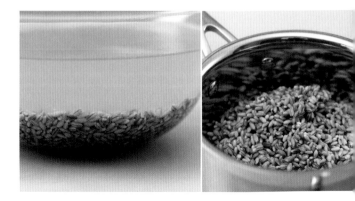

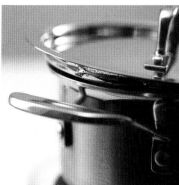
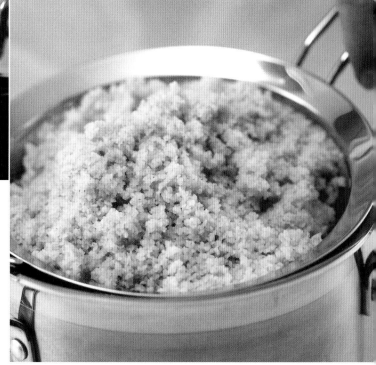

Bulgur wheat

A form of cracked wheat, bulgur has had some or all of the bran removed. It is good served as an accompaniment or used in salads. It is pre-boiled during manufacturing and may be boiled, steamed or soaked.

Simmering bulgur Put the bulgur in a pan and add water to cover by about 2.5cm (1in). Bring to the boil, then simmer for 10–15 minutes until just tender. Drain well.

Steaming bulgur Place the bulgur in a steamer lined with a clean teatowel and steam over boiling water for 20 minutes or until the grains are soft.

Soaking bulgur Put the bulgur in a deep bowl. Cover with hot water and mix with a fork. Leave to steep for 20 minutes, checking to make sure there is enough water. Drain and fluff up with a fork.

Quantities

Allow 50–75g (2–3oz) raw grain per person. Or, if measuring by volume, allow 50–75ml (2–2¹/₂fl oz).

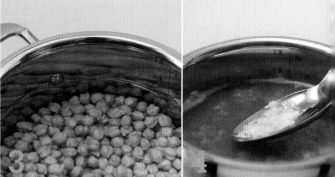

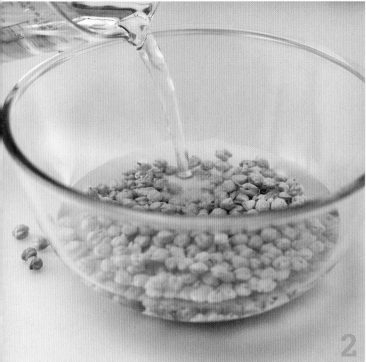

Cooking dried beans

1   Pick through the beans to remove any grit or small stones.

2   Put the beans in a bowl or pan and pour over cold water to cover generously. Leave to soak for at least 8 hours, then drain. (If you are in a hurry, pour boiling water over the beans and leave them to cool in the water for 1–2 hours.)

3   Put the soaked beans in a large pan and add water to cover by at least 5cm (2in). Bring to the boil and boil rapidly for 10 minutes.

4   Skim off the scum that rises to the top, turn down the heat and leave to simmer until the beans are soft inside. They should be tender but not falling apart. Check the water periodically to make sure there's enough to keep the beans well covered. Drain well. If using in a salad, allow to cool completely.

Using beans and lentils

Many dried beans and peas need to be soaked overnight before cooking. However, lentils do not need soaking and are quicker to cook. Quicker still are canned beans: they are ready to use, but should be drained in a sieve and rinsed in cold water first.

Cooking times

Times vary for different dried beans, peas and lentils. Older beans will take longer to cook, so use them within their 'best before' date.

Chickpeas	1–2 hours
Red kidney, cannellini, borlotti, butter, flageolet beans	1–3 hours
Red lentils	20 minutes
Green lentils	30–40 minutes

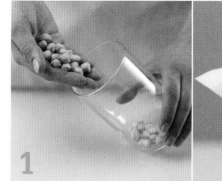

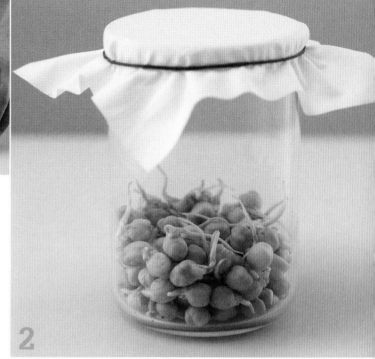

Sprouting beans

Mung beans, chickpeas, green or Puy lentils and alfalfa are popular for home sprouting and are good in salads and stir-fries. You will only need about 3 tbsp beans to sprout at one time.

1 Pick through the beans to remove any grit or stones, then soak in cold water for at least 8 hours. Drain and place in a clean (preferably sterilised) jar. Cover the top with a dampened piece of clean cloth, secure and leave in a warm, dark place.

2 Rinse the sprouting beans twice a day. The sprouts can be eaten when there is about 1cm ($^{1}/_{2}$in) of growth, or they can be left to grow for a day or two longer. When they are sprouted, leave the jar on a sunny windowsill for about 3 hours – this will improve both their flavour and their nutrients. Then rinse and dry them well. They can be kept for about three days in the refrigerator. Always rinse the beans well before using them.

Storing beans

Always store dried beans, peas and lentils in airtight containers in a cool, dry place. Use within 1 year – or check the 'best before' date. Do not mix old and new beans because they will take different times to cook.

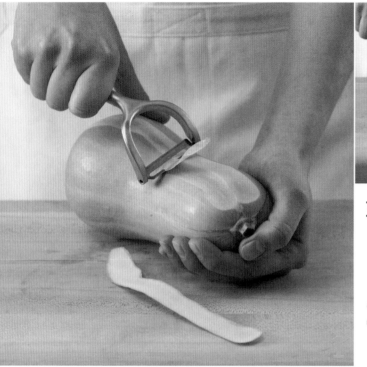

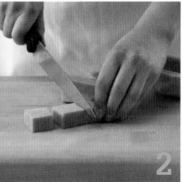

Peeling and cutting squash

1 For steaming, baking or roasting, keep the chunks fairly large – at least 2.5cm (1in) thick. Peel with a swivel-headed peeler or a cook's knife.

2 Halve the squash, then use a knife to cut through some of the fibrous mass connecting the seeds with the wall of the central cavity. Scoop out the seeds and fibres with a spoon, then cut the flesh into pieces.

Preparing vegetables

Vegetables are a vital part of a healthy diet. Here are some preparation methods for everyday and more unusual varieties.

Cooking squash in the skin

1 Wash the squash, then cut in half or quarters.

2 Use a knife to cut through some of the fibrous mass connecting the seeds with the wall of the central cavity, then use a spoon to scoop out the seeds and fibres.

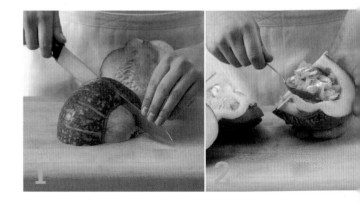

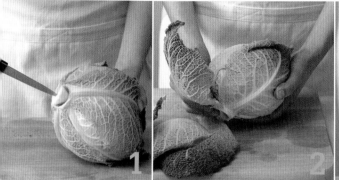

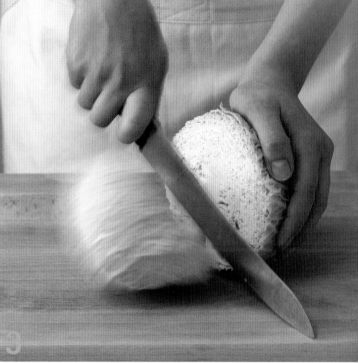

Cabbage

The crinkly leaved Savoy cabbage may need more washing than other varieties, because its open leaves catch dirt more easily than the tightly packed white and red cabbage. The following method is suitable for all cabbages.

1   Pick off any of the outer leaves that are dry, tough or discoloured. Cut off the base and, using a small sharp knife, cut out as much as possible of the tough inner core in a single cone-shaped piece.

2   If you need whole cabbage leaves, peel them off one by one. As you work your way down, you will need to cut out more of the core.

3   If you are cooking the cabbage in wedges, cut it in half lengthways, then cut the pieces into wedges of the required size.

Shredding cabbage

If you want fine shreds, you can make them easily on the shredding disc of a food processor. To shred by hand, cut the cabbage into quarters before slicing with a large cook's knife.

Cauliflower

First cut off the base and remove the outer leaves, then cut out the tough inner core in a cone-shaped piece as for cabbage (above). Cut off the florets in the same way as for broccoli (right). Don't cut away too much of the stalk or the florets will fall apart.

Broccoli

1   Slice off the end of the stalk and cut 1cm ($\frac{1}{2}$in) below the florets. Cut the broccoli head in half.

2   Peel the thick, woody skin from the stalks and slice the stalks in half or quarters lengthways. Cut off equal-sized florets with a small knife. If the florets are very large, or if you want them for a stir-fry, you can halve them by cutting lengthways through the stalk and pulling the two halves apart.

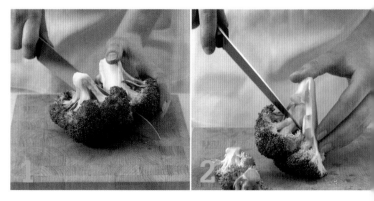

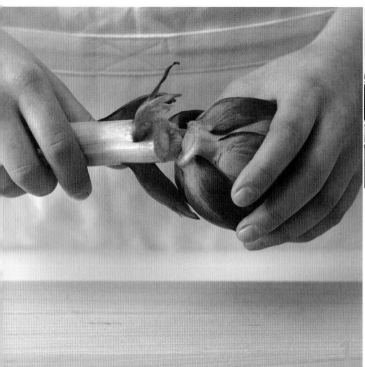

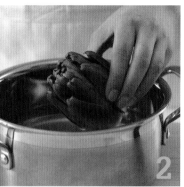

Whole artichokes

1 Snap off the stalk so that it's level with the base of the leaves. Tear off any dry or discoloured leaves, and rinse in cold water.

2 Put the artichokes in a pan of salted boiling water with 1 tsp lemon juice and weigh them down with a bowl so that they are completely covered. Boil for 40–45 minutes until an outer leaf pulls off easily.

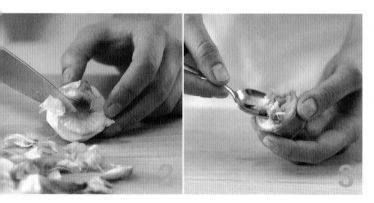

Artichoke hearts

1 Heat a pan of salted water with 1 tbsp lemon juice per 1 litre (1³/₄ pints) of water.

2 Remove the stalk and outer leaves, then cut off the remaining leaves and trim away the green parts from the base. Rub with lemon juice and cook for 15–20 minutes until tender.

3 Drain, then scoop out the choke.

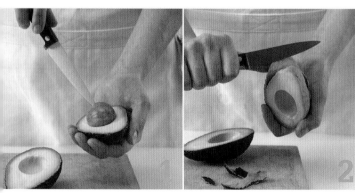

Avocados

1 Prepare avocados just before serving because their flesh discolours quickly once exposed to air. Halve the avocado lengthways and twist the two halves apart. Tap the stone with a sharp knife, then twist to remove the stone.

2 Run a knife between the flesh and skin and pull away. Slice the flesh.

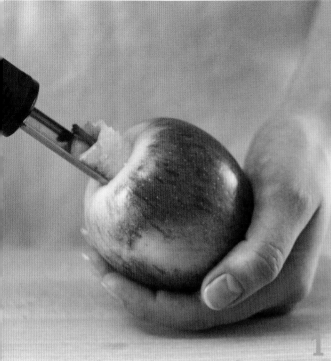

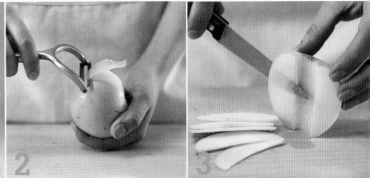

Apples

1 To core an apple, push an apple corer straight through the apple from the stem to the base. Remove the core and use a small sharp knife to pick out any stray seeds or seed casings.

2 To peel, hold the fruit in one hand and run a swivel-headed peeler under the skin, starting from the stem end and moving around the fruit, taking off the skin until you reach the base.

3 To slice, halve the cored apple. For flat slices, hold the apple cut side down and slice with the knife blade at right angles to the hollow left by the core. For crescent-shaped slices, stand the fruit on its end and cut slices into the hollow as if you were slicing a pie.

Preserving colour

Apples are easy to work with because they are very firm-fleshed, but their flesh turns brown when exposed to air and starts to discolour quickly. Toss with lemon juice if you are not going to use the prepared fruit immediately.

Preparing fruit

Nutritionally, fruit is important – both as a source of dietary fibre and of minerals and vitamins, especially vitamin C. Some varieties, especially apricots, mangoes and peaches, also provide vitamin A in the form of carotene. All fruits provide some energy, in the form of fructose (or fruit sugar), but most varieties are very low in fat and therefore low in calories. A few simple techniques can make preparing both familiar and not-so-familiar fruits quick and easy.

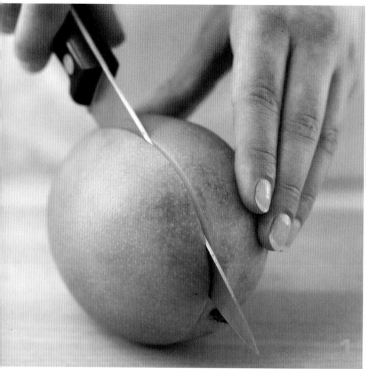

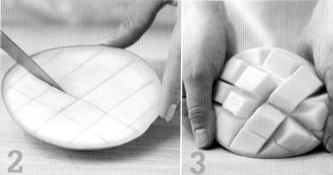

Mangoes

1   Cut a slice to one side of the stone in the centre. Repeat on the other side.

2   Cut parallel lines into the flesh of one slice, almost to the skin. Cut another set of lines to cut the flesh into squares.

3   Press on the skin side to turn the fruit inside out, so that the flesh is thrust outwards. Cut off the chunks as close as possible to the skin. Repeat with the other half.

Papaya

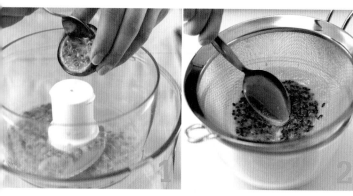

1   If using in a salad, peel the fruit using a swivel-headed peeler, then gently cut in half using a sharp knife. Remove the seeds using a teaspoon and slice the flesh, or cut into cubes.

2   If serving on its own, halve the fruit lengthways using a sharp knife, then use a teaspoon to scoop out the shiny black seeds and fibres inside the cavity.

Passion fruit

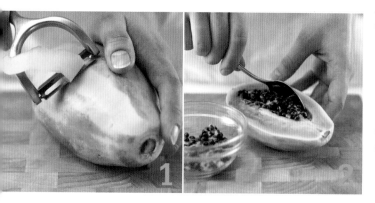

1   The seeds are edible but if you want the fruit for a purée, you will need to sieve them. Halve the passion fruit and scoop the seeds and pulp into a food processor or blender. Process for 30 seconds, until the mixture looks soupy.

2   Pour into a sieve over a bowl, and press down hard on the pulp with the back of a spoon to release the juice.

Pineapples

1 Cut off the base and crown of the pineapple, and stand the fruit on a chopping board.

2 Using a medium-sized knife, peel away a section of skin, going just deep enough to remove all or most of the hard, inedible 'eyes' on the skin. Repeat all the way around.

3 Use a small knife to cut out any remaining traces of the eyes.

4 Cut the peeled pineapple into slices.

5 You can buy special tools for coring pineapples but a 7.5cm (3in) biscuit cutter or an apple corer works just as well. Place the biscuit cutter directly over the core and press down firmly. If using an apple corer, cut out the core in pieces, as it will be too wide to remove in one piece.

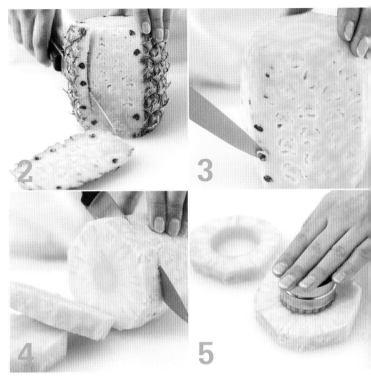

Pomegranate

1 Cut off the base of the fruit, trying not to cut into the cells containing seeds, and make four shallow cuts into the skin with a small sharp knife. Break the pomegranate in half, and then into quarters.

2 Bend the skin of each quarter backwards to push the seeds out into a bowl. Remove any left behind with a teaspoon. Remove and discard any of the bitter pith that remains on the seeds.

3 To extract the juice from the seeds, pound them in a mortar with a pestle.

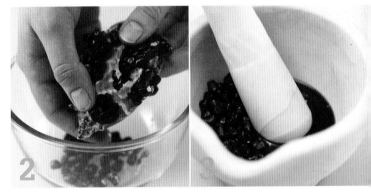

Cook's Tips

Do not press hard when extracting the juice, or it will have a bitter taste.
Take care: the juice stains.

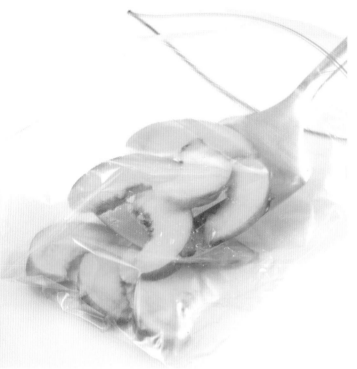

Food storage and hygiene

Storing food properly and preparing it in a hygienic way is important to ensure that food remains as nutritious and flavourful as possible, and to reduce the risk of food poisoning.

Hygiene

When you are preparing food, always follow these important guidelines:

Wash your hands thoroughly before handling food and again between handling different types of food, such as raw and cooked meat and poultry. If you have any cuts or grazes on your hands, be sure to keep them covered with a waterproof plaster.

Wash down worksurfaces regularly with a mild detergent solution or multi-surface cleaner.

Use a dishwasher if available. Otherwise, wear rubber gloves for washing-up, so that the water temperature can be hotter than unprotected hands can bear. Change drying-up cloths and cleaning cloths regularly. Note that leaving dishes to drain is more hygienic than drying them with a teatowel.

Keep raw and cooked foods separate, especially meat, fish and poultry. Wash kitchen utensils in between preparing raw and cooked foods. Never put cooked or ready-to-eat foods directly on to a surface which has just had raw fish, meat or poultry on it.

Keep pets out of the kitchen if possible; or make sure they stay away from worksurfaces. Never allow animals on to worksurfaces.

Shopping

Always choose fresh ingredients in prime condition from stores and markets that have a regular turnover of stock to ensure you buy the freshest produce possible.

Make sure items are within their 'best before' or 'use by' date. (Foods with a longer shelf life have a 'best before' date; more perishable items have a 'use by' date.)

Pack frozen and chilled items in an insulated cool bag at the check-out and put them into the freezer or refrigerator as soon as you get home.

During warm weather in particular, buy perishable foods just before you return home. When packing items at the check-out, sort them according to where you will store them when you get home – the refrigerator, freezer, storecupboard, vegetable rack, fruit bowl, etc. This will make unpacking easier – and quicker.

The storecupboard

Although storecupboard ingredients will generally last a long time, correct storage is important:

Always check packaging for storage advice – even with familiar foods, because storage requirements may change if additives, sugar or salt have been reduced. Check storecupboard foods for their 'best before' or 'use by' date and do not use them if the date has passed.

Keep all food cupboards scrupulously clean and make sure food containers and packets are properly sealed.

Once opened, treat canned foods as though fresh. Always transfer the contents to a clean container, cover and keep in the refrigerator. Similarly, jars, sauce bottles and cartons should be kept chilled after opening. (Check the label for safe storage times after opening.)

Transfer dry goods such as sugar, rice and pasta to moisture-proof containers. When supplies are used up, wash the container well and thoroughly dry before refilling with new supplies.

Store oils in a dark cupboard away from any heat source as heat and light can make them turn rancid and affect their colour. For the same reason, buy olive oil in dark green bottles.

Store vinegars in a cool place; they can turn bad in a warm environment.

Store dried herbs, spices and flavourings in a cool, dark cupboard or in dark jars. Buy in small quantities as their flavour will not last indefinitely.

Store flours and sugars in airtight containers.

Refrigerator storage

Fresh food needs to be stored in the cool temperature of the refrigerator to keep it in good condition and discourage the growth of harmful bacteria. Store day-to-day perishable items, such as opened jams and jellies, mayonnaise and bottled sauces, in the refrigerator along with eggs and dairy products, fruit juices, bacon, fresh and cooked meat (on separate shelves), and salads and vegetables (except potatoes, which don't suit being stored in the cold). A refrigerator should be kept at an operating temperature of 4–5°C.

It is worth investing in a refrigerator thermometer to ensure the correct temperature is maintained. To ensure your refrigerator is functioning effectively for safe food storage, follow these guidelines:

To avoid bacterial cross-contamination, store cooked and raw foods on separate shelves, putting cooked foods on the top shelf. Ensure that all items are well wrapped.

Never put hot food into the refrigerator, as this will cause the internal temperature of the refrigerator to rise.

Avoid overfilling the refrigerator, as this restricts the circulation of air and prevents the appliance from working properly.

It can take some time for the refrigerator to return to the correct operating temperature once the door has been opened, so don't leave it open any longer than is necessary.

Clean the refrigerator regularly, using a specially formulated germicidal refrigerator cleaner. Alternatively, use a weak solution of bicarbonate of soda: 1 tbsp to 1 litre (1³/₄ pints) water.

If your refrigerator doesn't have an automatic defrost facility, defrost regularly.

Maximum refrigerator storage times

For pre-packed foods, always adhere to the 'use by' date on the packet. For other foods the following storage times should apply, providing the food is in prime condition when it goes into the refrigerator and that your refrigerator is in good working order:

Vegetables and Fruit

Green vegetables	3–4 days
Salad leaves	2–3 days
Hard and stone fruit	3–7 days
Soft fruit	1–2 days

Dairy Food

Cheese, hard	1 week
Cheese, soft	2–3 days
Eggs	1 week
Milk	4–5 days

Fish

Fish	1 day
Shellfish	1 day

Raw Meat

Bacon	7 days
Game	2 days
Joints	3 days
Minced meat	1 day
Offal	1 day
Poultry	2 days
Raw sliced meat	2 days
Sausages	3 days

Cooked Meat

Joints	3 days
Casseroles/stews	2 days
Pies	2 days
Sliced meat	2 days
Ham	2 days
Ham, vacuum-packed (or according to the instructions on the packet)	1–2 weeks

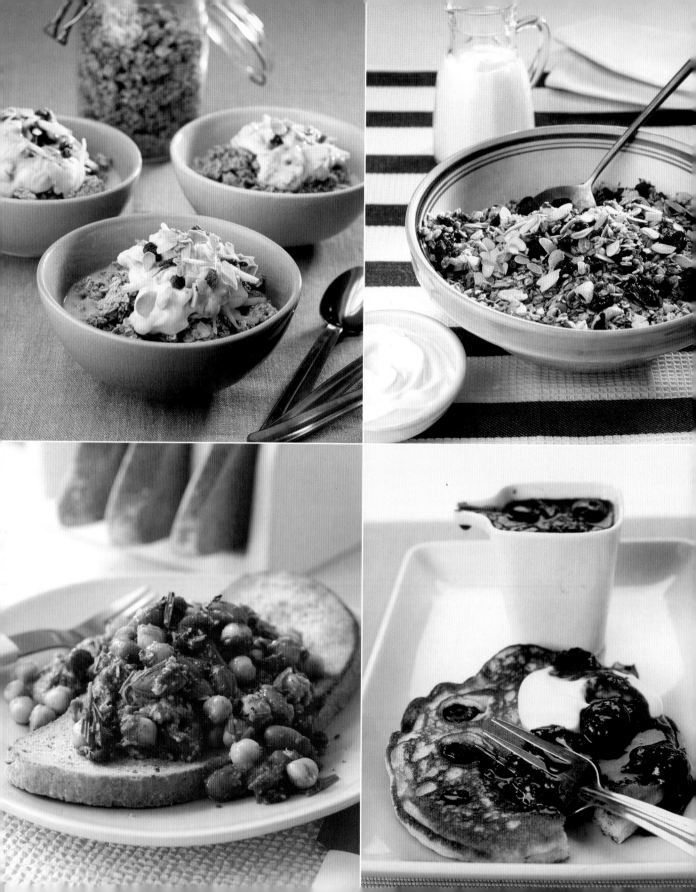

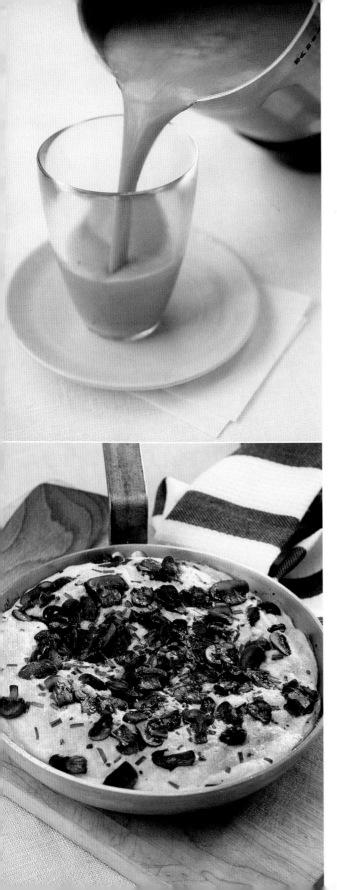

1

Start the Day

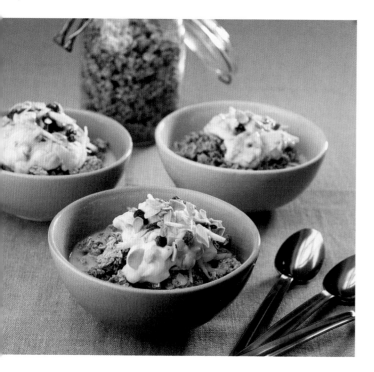

Try Something Different

Use pears instead of apples.
Replace the sultanas with dried cranberries.

Apple and Almond Yogurt

500g (1lb 2oz) natural yogurt

50g (2oz) each flaked almonds and sultanas

2 apples

1   Put the yogurt in a bowl and add the almonds and sultanas.

2   Grate the apples, add to the bowl and mix together. Chill in the fridge overnight. Use as a topping for breakfast cereal or serve as a snack.

Serves 4	EASY		NUTRITIONAL INFORMATION	
	Preparation Time 5 minutes, plus overnight chilling		**Per Serving** 192 calories, 8g fat (of which 1g saturates), 22g carbohydrate, 0.3g salt	Vegetarian Gluten free

300g (11oz) rolled oats

50g (2oz) each chopped Brazil nuts, flaked almonds, wheatgerm or rye flakes, and sunflower seeds

25g (1oz) sesame seeds

100ml (3½fl oz) sunflower oil

3 tbsp runny honey

100g (3½oz) each raisins and dried cranberries

Granola
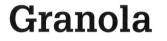

1 Preheat the oven to 140°C (120°C fan oven) mark 1. Put the oats, nuts, wheatgerm or rye flakes, and all the seeds in a bowl. Gently heat the oil and honey in a pan. Pour over the oats and stir to combine. Spread on a shallow baking tray and cook in the oven for 1 hour or until golden, stirring once. Leave to cool.

2 Transfer to a bowl and stir in the dried fruit. Store in an airtight container – the granola will keep for up to a week. Serve with milk or yogurt.

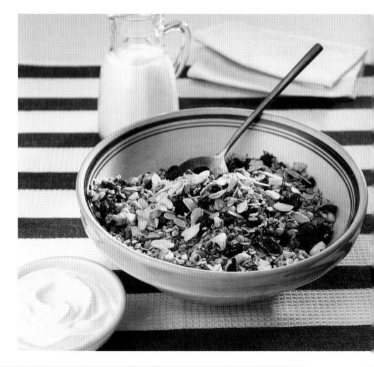

EASY		NUTRITIONAL INFORMATION		Makes
Preparation Time 5 minutes	**Cooking Time** 1 hour 5 minutes	**Per Serving** 254 calories, 14g fat (of which 2g saturates), 29g carbohydrate, 0g salt	Vegetarian Dairy free	**15** servings

Porridge with Dried Fruit

200g (7oz) rolled oats

400ml (14fl oz) milk, plus extra to serve

75g (3oz) mixture of chopped dried figs, apricots and raisins

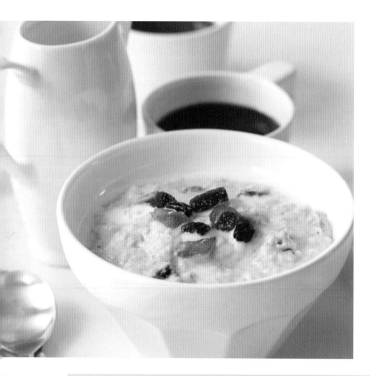

1 Put the oats into a large pan and add the milk and 400ml (14fl oz) water. Stir in the chopped dried figs, apricots and raisins and heat gently, stirring until the porridge thickens and the oats are cooked.

2 Divide among four bowls and serve with a splash of milk.

Serves 4	EASY		NUTRITIONAL INFORMATION	
	Preparation Time 5 minutes	Cooking Time 5 minutes	Per Serving 280 calories, 6g fat (of which 1g saturates), 49g carbohydrate, 0.2g salt	Vegetarian

Try Something Different

Instead of blueberries and lemon, use 100g (3½oz) chopped ready-to-eat dried apricots and 2 tsp grated fresh root ginger.

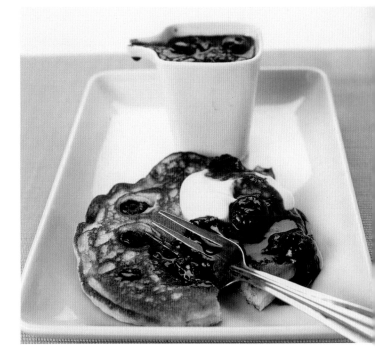

Lemon and Blueberry Pancakes

125g (4oz) wholemeal plain flour
1 tsp baking powder
¼ tsp bicarbonate of soda
2 tbsp golden caster sugar
finely grated zest of 1 unwaxed lemon
125g (4oz) natural yogurt
2 tbsp milk
2 medium eggs
40g (1½oz) butter
100g (3½oz) blueberries
1 tsp sunflower oil
natural yogurt and fruit compote to serve

1 Sift the flour, baking powder and bicarbonate of soda into a bowl, tipping in the contents left in the sieve. Add the sugar and lemon zest. Pour in the yogurt and milk. Break the eggs into the mixture and whisk together.

2 Melt 25g (1oz) butter in a pan, add to the bowl with the blueberries, then stir everything together.

3 Heat a dot of butter with the sunflower oil in a frying pan over a medium heat until hot. Add four large spoonfuls of the mixture to the pan to make four pancakes. After about 2 minutes, flip over and cook for 1–2 minutes. Repeat with the remaining mixture, adding a dot more butter each time.

4 Serve with natural yogurt and some fruit compote.

EASY		NUTRITIONAL INFORMATION		Serves
Preparation Time 15 minutes	**Cooking Time** 10–15 minutes	**Per Serving** 290 calories, 13g fat (of which 6g saturates), 39g carbohydrate, 0.6g salt	Vegetarian	**4**

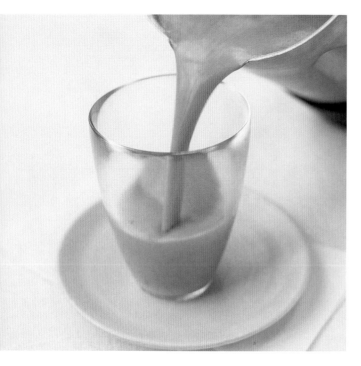

Cook's Tip

If you're on a dairy-free diet or are looking for an alternative to milk-based products, swap the yogurt for soya yogurt. Soya is a good source of essential omega-3 and omega-6 fatty acids, and can help to lower cholesterol.

Cranberry and Mango Smoothie

1 ripe mango, stone removed
250ml (9fl oz) cranberry juice
150g (5oz) natural yogurt

1 Peel and roughly chop the mango and put into a blender with the cranberry juice. Blend for 1 minute.

2 Add the yogurt and blend until smooth, then serve.

Serves 2	EASY	NUTRITIONAL INFORMATION	
	Preparation Time 5 minutes	**Per Serving** 133 calories, 1g fat (of which trace saturates), 29g carbohydrate, 0.2g salt	Vegetarian Gluten free

Try Something Different

Fresh strawberries or peaches would taste great instead of the frozen summer fruits.

Summer Berry Smoothie

2 large, ripe bananas, about 450g (1lb), peeled and chopped

150g (5oz) natural yogurt

150ml (¼ pint) spring water

500g (1lb 2oz) frozen summer fruits

1 Put the bananas, yogurt and spring water into a food processor or blender and whiz until smooth. Add the frozen berries and whiz to a purée.

2 Sieve the mixture, using the back of a ladle to press it through. Pour into glasses and serve.

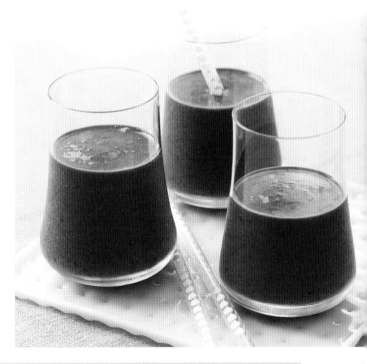

EASY	NUTRITIONAL INFORMATION		Serves
Preparation Time 10 minutes	**Per Serving** 107 calories, trace fat, 24g carbohydrate, 0.1g salt	Vegetarian Gluten free	**6**

Mushroom Soufflé Omelette

50g (2oz) small chestnut mushrooms, sliced

2 tbsp low-fat crème fraîche

2 medium eggs, separated

15g (½oz) butter

5 chives, roughly chopped

salt and ground black pepper

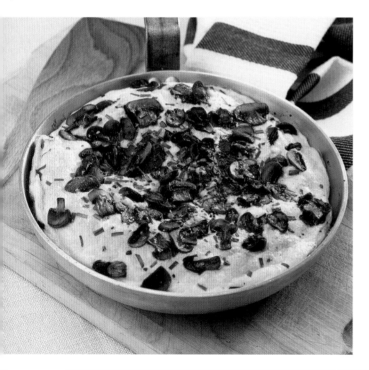

1 Heat a small, non-stick frying pan for 30 seconds. Add the mushrooms and cook, stirring, for 3 minutes to brown slightly, then stir in the crème fraîche and turn off the heat.

2 Lightly beat the egg yolks in a bowl, add 2 tbsp cold water and season with salt and pepper.

3 In a separate bowl, whisk the egg whites until stiff but not dry. Fold, very gently, into the egg yolks. Do not overmix. Heat an 18cm (7in) non-stick frying pan and melt the butter. Add the egg mixture, tilting the pan in all directions so the base is covered. Cook over a medium heat for 3 minutes or until the underside is golden brown.

4 Meanwhile, preheat the grill to medium. Gently reheat the mushrooms and add the chives. Put the omelette under the grill for 1 minute or until the surface is just firm and puffy. Tip the mushroom mixture on top. Run a spatula around and underneath the omelette to loosen it, then carefully fold it and turn on to a plate.

Serves 1	EASY		NUTRITIONAL INFORMATION	
	Preparation Time 5 minutes	**Cooking Time** 7–10 minutes	**Per Serving** 314 calories, 28g fat (of which 14g saturates), 2g carbohydrate, 0.6g salt	Vegetarian Gluten free

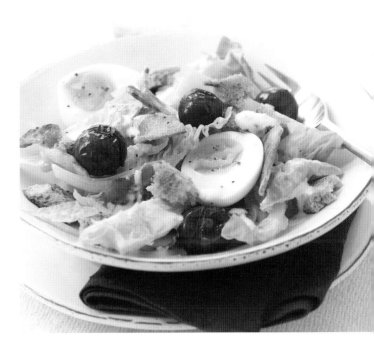

Bacon and Egg Salad

4 eggs

250g (9oz) rindless smoked bacon

150g (5oz) cherry tomatoes

2 slices thick-cut sourdough bread, with crusts removed

2 tbsp mayonnaise

juice of ½ lemon

25g (1oz) Parmesan, freshly grated

2 Little Gem lettuces

ground black pepper

1 Heat a pan of water until simmering, add the eggs and boil for 6 minutes. Cool completely under cold water, peel and set aside.

2 Meanwhile, heat a griddle pan, then fry the bacon for 5 minutes until crisp. Remove from the pan, chop into large pieces and leave to cool.

3 Add the tomatoes and bread to the pan and fry for 2–3 minutes until the bread is crisp and the tomatoes are starting to char. Remove from the heat, chop the bread into bite-sized croûtons and set aside.

4 To make the dressing, put the mayonnaise in a bowl and squeeze in the lemon juice. Add the Parmesan, mix, then season with pepper.

5 Separate the lettuce leaves and put in a large bowl. Add the bacon, tomatoes and croûtons, toss lightly, then divide among four serving plates. Cut the eggs in half and add one egg to each plate. Drizzle the dressing over.

EASY		NUTRITIONAL INFORMATION	Serves
Preparation Time 10 minutes	**Cooking Time** 10 minutes	**Per Serving** 360 calories, 27g fat (of which 8g saturates), 9g carbohydrate, 3.1g salt	**4**

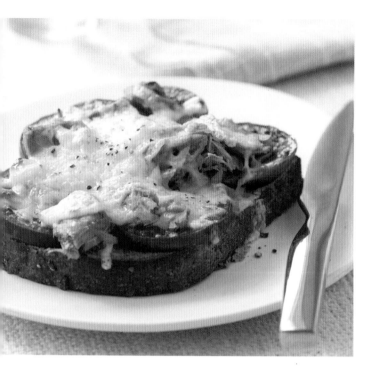

Try Something Different

Instead of tuna use a 120g can sardines or mackerel.

Tuna Melt

2 slices Granary, sourdough or wholemeal bread

2 tomatoes, sliced

75g (3oz) canned tuna in brine, drained

2 tbsp mayonnaise

50g (2oz) Cheddar or Red Leicester cheese, grated

dash of Worcestershire sauce

1 Preheat the grill. Toast the bread on one side then turn it over.

2 Divide the sliced tomatoes between the two slices of bread, then add the tuna.

3 Spread the mayonnaise over the tuna and cover with the grated cheese. Sprinkle a dash of Worcestershire sauce on each. Grill until the cheese is golden and bubbling.

Serves 2	EASY		NUTRITIONAL INFORMATION
	Preparation Time 5 minutes	**Cooking Time** 5 minutes	**Per Serving** 390 calories, 21g fat (of which 8g saturates), 30g carbohydrate, 1.7g salt

1 tbsp olive oil

2 garlic cloves, finely sliced

400g can borlotti or cannellini beans, drained and rinsed

400g can chickpeas, drained and rinsed

400g can chopped tomatoes

2 rosemary sprigs

4 slices sourdough or Granary bread

25g (1oz) Parmesan

Low-GI Beans on Toast

1 Heat the oil in a pan over a low heat, add the garlic and cook for 1 minute, stirring gently.

2 Add the beans and chickpeas to the pan with the tomatoes, and bring to the boil. Strip the leaves from the rosemary, then chop finely and add to the pan. Reduce the heat and simmer for 8–10 minutes until thickened.

3 Meanwhile, toast the bread and put on to plates. Grate the Parmesan into the bean mixture, stir once, then spoon over the bread. Serve immediately.

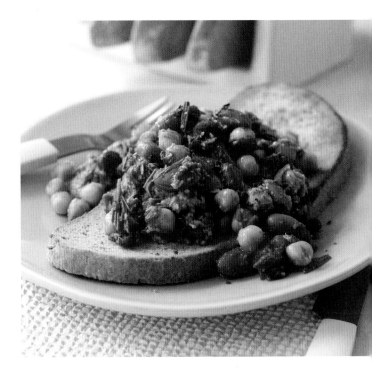

EASY		NUTRITIONAL INFORMATION		Serves
Preparation Time 5 minutes	**Cooking Time** 10 minutes	**Per Serving** 364 calories, 9g fat (of which 2g saturates), 55g carbohydrate, 2.1g salt	Vegetarian	**4**

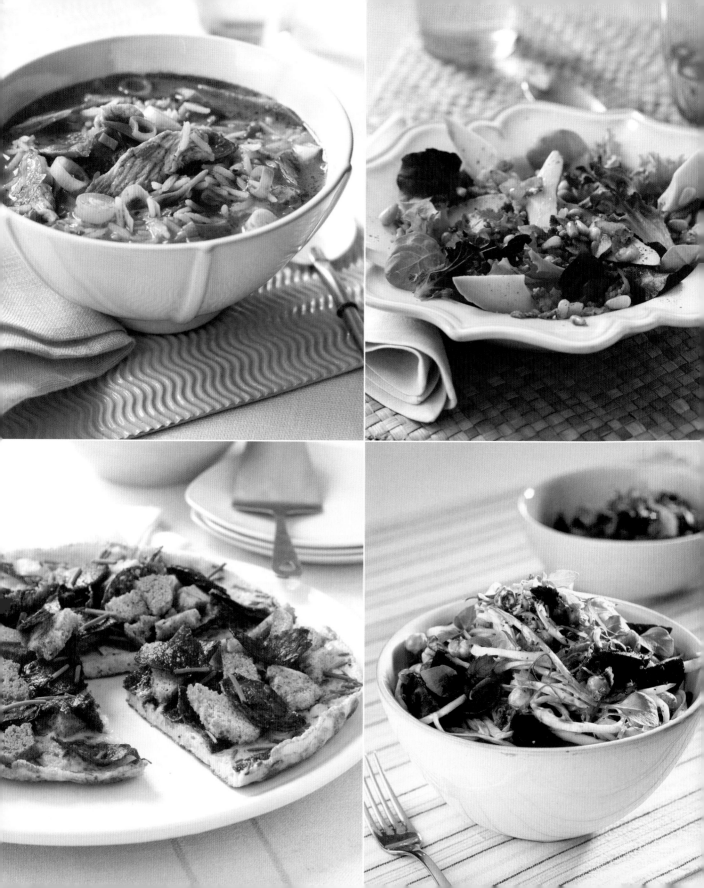

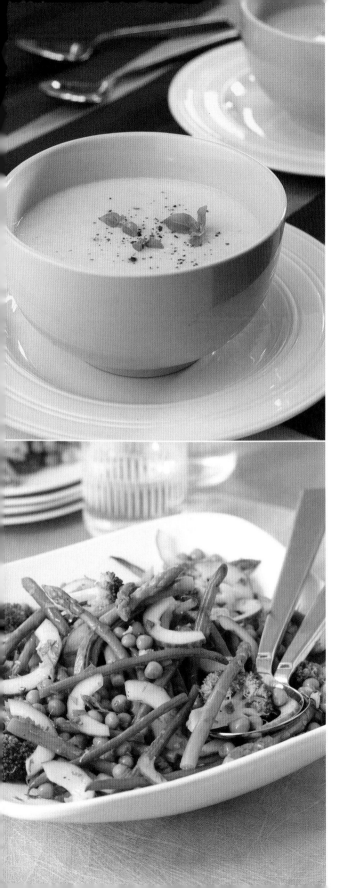

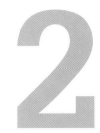

Soups, Salads and Quick Bites

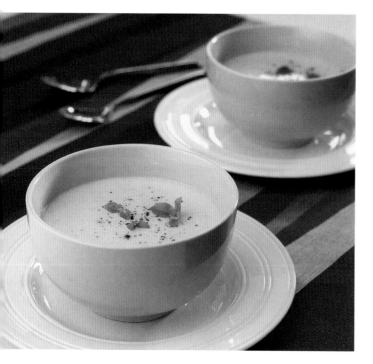

Try Something Different

Instead of celery use 500g (1lb 2oz) celeriac, peeled and diced. Replace the sage with 2 tsp chopped thyme.

Celery Soup

25g (1oz) butter
1 tbsp olive oil
1 medium leek, sliced
6 celery sticks, finely sliced
1 tbsp finely chopped sage
600ml (1 pint) hot chicken stock
300ml (½ pint) milk
salt and ground black pepper
basil sprigs to garnish

1 Melt the butter in a pan and add the oil. Add the leek and fry for 10–15 minutes until soft. Add the celery and sage and cook for 5 minutes to soften.

2 Add the hot chicken stock and milk to the pan, then season with salt and pepper, cover and bring to the boil. Reduce the heat and simmer for 10–15 minutes until the celery is tender.

3 Leave to cool a little, then whiz in a food processor or blender. Return the soup to the pan, reheat gently and season with salt and pepper. Divide among four warmed bowls and garnish with basil.

Serves 4	EASY		NUTRITIONAL INFORMATION	
	Preparation Time 10 minutes	Cooking Time 30–40 minutes	Per Serving 123 calories, 10g fat (of which 5g saturates), 6g carbohydrate, 0.8g salt	Gluten free

Freezing Tip

Freeze the soup at step 3 for up to one month.
To use Thaw overnight in the fridge. Reheat gently and simmer for 5 minutes.

1 tbsp olive oil

1 large onion, chopped

1 tbsp coriander seeds

900g (2lb) carrots, roughly chopped

2 medium sweet potatoes, roughly chopped

2 litres (3½ pints) hot vegetable or chicken stock

2 tbsp white wine vinegar

2 tbsp chopped coriander, plus extra coriander leaves to garnish

4 tbsp half-fat crème fraîche

salt and ground black pepper

Carrot and Sweet Potato Soup

1 Heat the oil in a large pan, add the onion and coriander seeds and cook over a medium heat for 5 minutes. Add the carrots and sweet potatoes and cook for a further 5 minutes.

2 Add the stock and bring the soup to the boil. Reduce the heat and leave to simmer for 25 minutes. Leave to cool slightly, then whiz in a blender until slightly chunky. Add the wine vinegar and season with salt and pepper.

3 Pour the soup into a clean pan, stir in the chopped coriander and reheat gently.

4 Drizzle over the crème fraîche and sprinkle on the coriander leaves. Serve in warmed bowls.

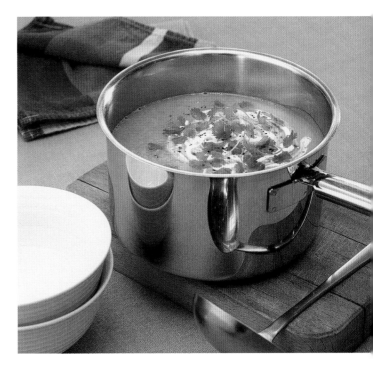

EASY		NUTRITIONAL INFORMATION		Serves
Preparation Time 15 minutes	**Cooking Time** 45 minutes	**Per Serving** 120 calories, 3g fat (of which 1g saturates), 22g carbohydrate, 0.7g salt	Vegetarian Gluten free	**8**

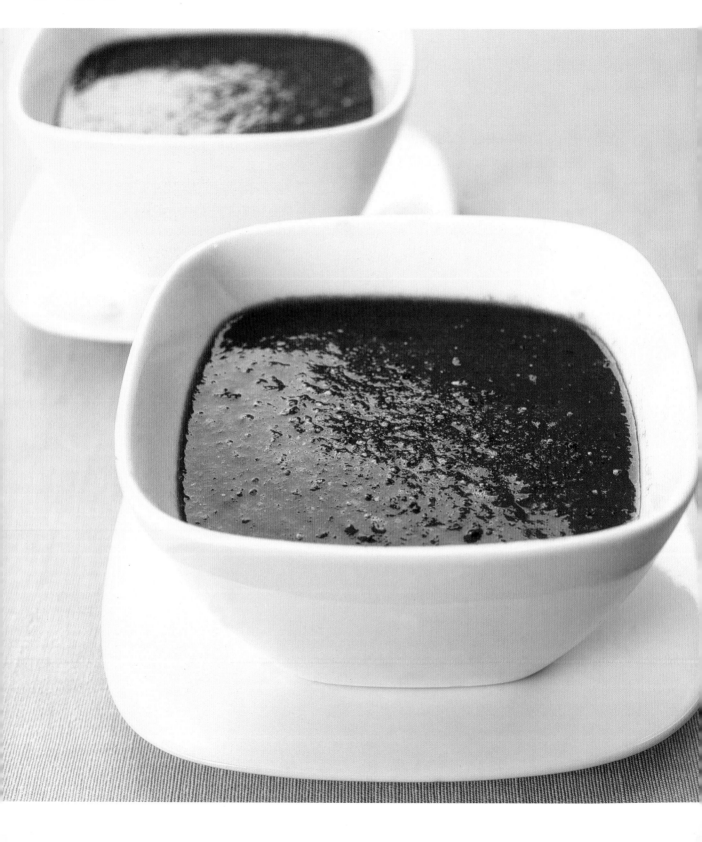

Tomato, Pepper and Orange Soup

3 rosemary sprigs
400g (14oz) jar roasted red peppers, drained
2 tsp golden caster sugar
1 litre (1¾ pints) tomato juice
4 very ripe plum tomatoes
300ml (½ pint) hot chicken stock
450ml (¾ pint) freshly squeezed orange juice
ground black pepper

1 Pull the leaves from the rosemary sprigs and discard the twiggy stalks. Put the leaves into a food processor or blender, add the peppers, sugar, half the tomato juice and the plum tomatoes and whiz together until slightly chunky.

2 Sieve the mixture into a pan and stir in the stock, orange juice and the remaining tomato juice. Bring to the boil and simmer gently for about 10 minutes. Season with plenty of pepper to serve.

Try Something Different

Instead of rosemary use a small handful of fresh coriander and add a dash or two of Tabasco before serving.

EASY		NUTRITIONAL INFORMATION		Serves
Preparation Time 15 minutes	**Cooking Time** 12 minutes	**Per Serving** 136 calories, 1g fat (of which trace saturates), 30g carbohydrate, 1.8g salt	Gluten free Dairy free	**4**

Fast Fish Soup

1 leek, finely sliced

4 fat garlic cloves, crushed

3 celery sticks, finely sliced

1 small fennel bulb, finely sliced

1 red chilli, seeded and finely chopped (see page 71)

3 tbsp olive oil

50ml (2fl oz) white wine

about 750g (1½lb) mixed fish and shellfish, such as haddock, monkfish, salmon, raw shelled prawns and cleaned mussels

4 medium tomatoes, chopped

20g (¾oz) fresh thyme, finely chopped

salt and ground black pepper

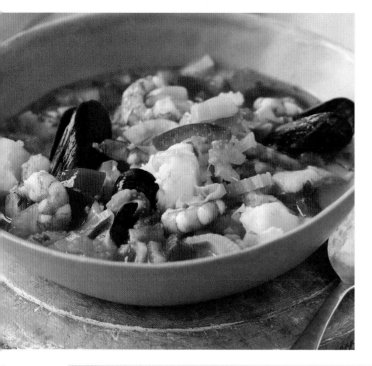

1 Put the leek in a large pan and add the garlic, celery, fennel, chilli and olive oil. Cook over a medium heat for 5 minutes or until the vegetables are soft and beginning to colour.

2 Stir in 1.1 litres (2 pints) boiling water and the wine. Bring to the boil, then simmer the soup, covered, for 5 minutes.

3 Meanwhile, cut the fish into large chunks. Add to the soup with the tomatoes and thyme. Continue simmering gently until the fish has just turned opaque. Add the prawns and simmer for 1 minute then add the mussels – if you're using them. As soon as all the mussels have opened, season the soup and ladle into warmed bowls. Discard any mussels that haven't opened.

Serves 4	EASY		NUTRITIONAL INFORMATION	
	Preparation Time 10 minutes	Cooking Time 15 minutes	Per Serving 269 calories, 10g fat (of which 2g saturates), 6g carbohydrate, 0.6g salt	Gluten free Dairy free

Cook's Tip

Red Thai curry paste is a hot chilli paste; if you prefer a milder version use green Thai curry paste.

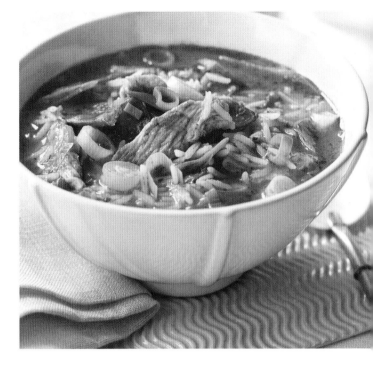

Hot and Sour Turkey Soup

1 tbsp vegetable oil

300g (11oz) turkey breasts, cut into strips

5cm (2in) piece fresh root ginger, grated

4 spring onions, finely sliced

1–2 tbsp red Thai curry paste

75g (3oz) basmati rice

1.1 litres (2 pints) weak hot chicken or vegetable stock, or boiling water

200g (7oz) mangetouts, sliced

juice of 1 lime

1   Heat the oil in a deep pan. Add the turkey and cook over a medium heat for 5 minutes until browned.

2   Add the ginger and spring onions. Cook for a further 2–3 minutes. Stir in the Thai curry paste and cook for 1–2 minutes to warm the spices.

3   Add the rice and stir to coat in the curry paste. Pour the hot stock into the pan, stir once and bring to the boil. Turn the heat down and leave to simmer, covered, for 20 minutes.

4   Add the mangetouts and simmer for 1–2 minutes, then stir in the lime juice before serving.

EASY		NUTRITIONAL INFORMATION		Serves
Preparation Time 25 minutes	**Cooking Time** 40 minutes	**Per Serving** 385 calories, 13g fat (of which 1g saturates), 39g carbohydrate, 1.6g salt	Gluten free Dairy free	**4**

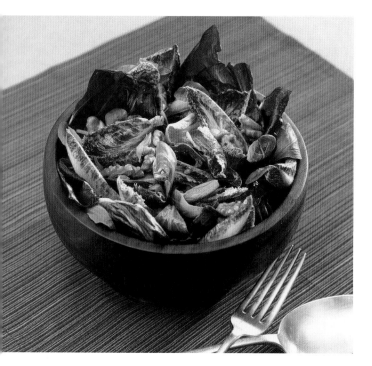

Try Something Different

Add orange segments for a really refreshing salad.

Winter Leaf Salad

75g (3oz) lamb's lettuce
1 small head radicchio
2 small red chicory
75g (3oz) walnuts, toasted and roughly chopped

For the dressing
2 tbsp white wine vinegar
2 tbsp walnut oil
4 tbsp olive oil
salt and ground black pepper

1 Put the dressing ingredients in a jam jar. Season with salt and pepper and shake well to mix.

2 Tear all the salad leaves into bite-sized pieces and put into a large bowl. Add the walnuts and toss to mix.

3 To serve, shake the dressing again, then pour it over the salad and toss well.

Serves 6	EASY	NUTRITIONAL INFORMATION	
	Preparation Time 10 minutes	**Per Serving** 196 calories, 20g fat (of which 2g saturates), 2g carbohydrate, 0.6g salt	Vegetarian Gluten free • Dairy free

Try Something Different

Yogurt dressing: mix together 5 tbsp natural yogurt with 1 tbsp each freshly chopped mint and chives and a small crushed garlic clove. Season with salt and pepper.

Tomato dressing: halve and seed 8 cherry tomatoes and cut into thin strips. Mix 1 tbsp balsamic vinegar with 3 tbsp olive oil, 2 tbsp freshly chopped tarragon, salt and pepper. Stir in the tomato and drizzle over the vegetables.

Summer Vegetable Salad

600g (1lb 5 oz) mixed green vegetables, such as green beans, peas, sugarsnap peas, trimmed asparagus, broad beans, broccoli

$^1/_4$ small cucumber, halved, seeded and sliced

2 tbsp freshly chopped flat-leafed parsley

For the dressing

1 tbsp white wine vinegar or sherry vinegar

1 tsp English mustard powder

3 tbsp extra virgin olive oil

salt and ground black pepper

1 Cook the beans in a large pan of salted boiling water for 3 minutes, then add all the other vegetables. Return the water to the boil and cook for a further 3–4 minutes. Drain well and put immediately into a bowl of ice-cold water.

2 Whisk all the dressing ingredients together and season with salt and pepper.

3 To serve, drain the vegetables and then toss in the dressing with the cucumber and parsley.

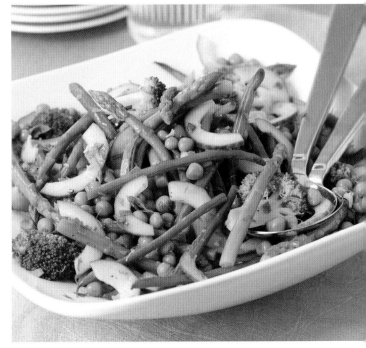

EASY		NUTRITIONAL INFORMATION		Serves
Preparation Time 10 minutes	**Cooking Time** 6–7 minutes	**Per Serving** 119 calories, 9g fat (of which 1g saturates), 4g carbohydrate, 0.6g salt	Vegetarian Gluten free • Dairy free	**4**

Spinach and Carrot Salad

350g (12oz) carrots, sliced

225g (8oz) green beans, trimmed

350g (12oz) baby leaf spinach

1 garlic clove, crushed

2 tsp each soy sauce and honey

1 tbsp cider vinegar

4 tbsp olive oil

ground black pepper

1 Cook the carrots in salted boiling water for 3–4 minutes, adding the beans for the last minute. Drain and rinse in cold water. Drain well, then put both in a bowl with the spinach.

2 Put the crushed garlic in a small bowl. Add the soy sauce, honey, cider vinegar and olive oil. Season with pepper and whisk together thoroughly. Pour some of the dressing over the carrot, bean and spinach mixture and toss together well. Serve the remaining dressing separately.

Try Something Different

Add a handful of sultanas or raisins, or lightly toasted sesame seeds.

Serves 4	EASY		NUTRITIONAL INFORMATION	
	Preparation Time 5 minutes	**Cooking Time** 4 minutes	**Per Serving** 173 calories, 12g fat (of which 2g saturates), 12g carbohydrate, 0.8g salt	Vegetarian Gluten free • Dairy free

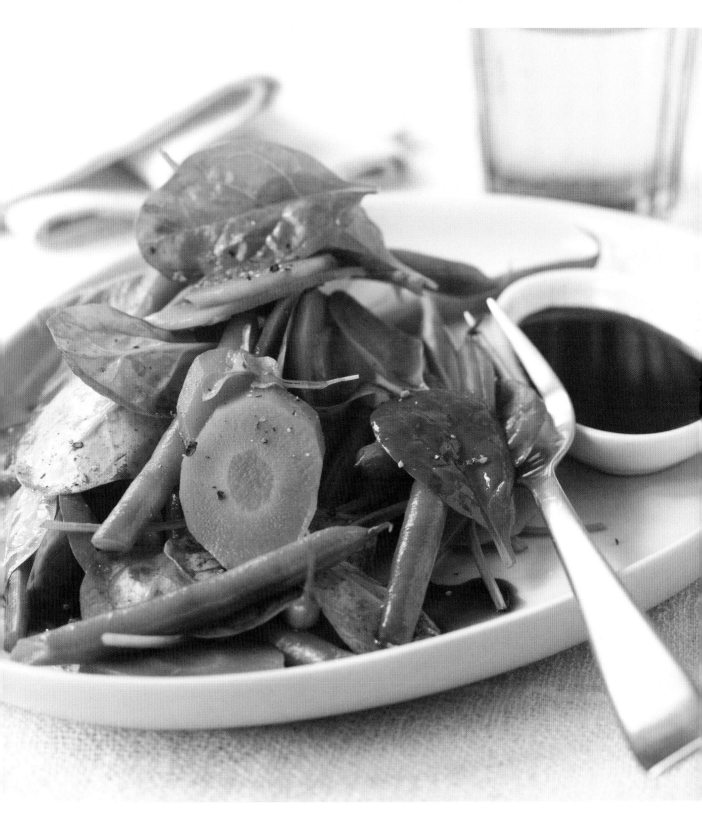

Try Something Different

Use parsley instead of basil, and add 4 finely chopped spring onions.
Scatter the salad with 2 tbsp lightly toasted pumpkin seeds or sunflower seeds.

250g (9oz) cooked beetroot (without vinegar), roughly chopped

400g can chickpeas, drained and rinsed

50g (2oz) sultanas

20g (³/₄oz) fresh basil

1 medium carrot, grated

¹/₂ small white cabbage, finely shredded

juice of ¹/₂ lemon

150g (5oz) Greek yogurt

20g (³/₄oz) fresh mint, finely chopped

2 tbsp extra virgin olive oil

salt and ground black pepper

Chickpea and Beetroot Salad

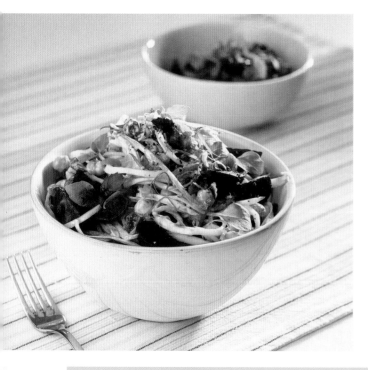

1 Put the beetroot and chickpeas in a large bowl. Add the sultanas, tear the basil and add, then add the carrot, cabbage and lemon juice.

2 Put the yogurt in a separate bowl. Add the mint and oil and season with salt and pepper. Spoon on to the salad and mix everything together. Serve immediately.

Serves 4	EASY		NUTRITIONAL INFORMATION	
	Preparation Time 15 minutes		**Per Serving** 266 calories, 12g fat (of which 3g saturates), 32g carbohydrate, 0.7g salt	Vegetarian Gluten free

▼ Pasta and Avocado Salad
▶ Spicy Swordfish (see page 101)
▶ Lemon Sorbet (see page 111)

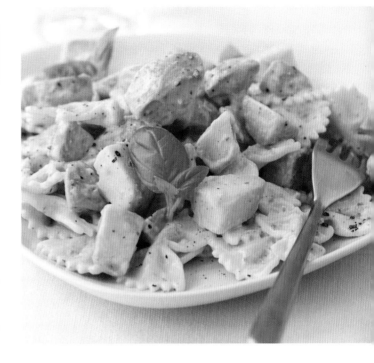

Pasta and Avocado Salad

2 tbsp mayonnaise

2 tbsp pesto

2 ripe avocados, halved, stoned, peeled and cut into cubes

225g (8oz) cooked pasta, cooled

a few basil leaves

1 Mix together the mayonnaise, pesto and avocado, then mix with the pasta. If the dressing is too thick, dilute with a little water (use the pasta cooking water if you have it).

2 Decorate with basil leaves and serve as a starter.

EASY	NUTRITIONAL INFORMATION		Serves
Preparation Time 5 minutes	**Per Serving** 313 calories, 26g fat (of which 5g saturates), 14g carbohydrate, 0.6g salt	Vegetarian Dairy free	**4**

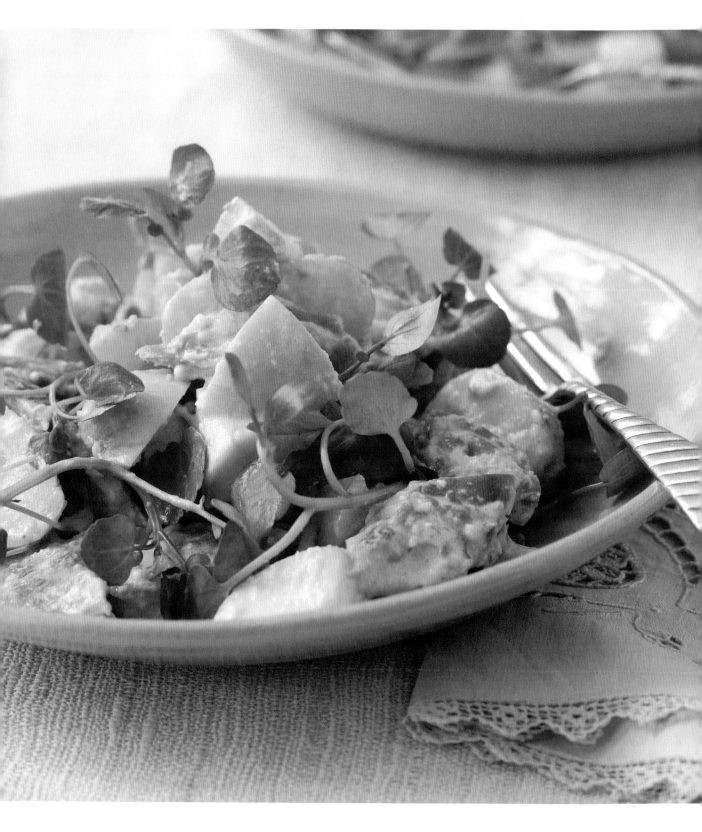

Smoked Mackerel with Potato and Horseradish Salad

350g (12oz) new potatoes, scrubbed
2 tbsp horseradish sauce
2 tbsp crème fraîche
1 tbsp lemon juice
4 tbsp olive oil
2 crisp apples
2 smoked mackerel fillets
100g (3½oz) watercress
ground black pepper

1 Cook the potatoes in a pan of salted boiling water for 15–20 minutes until tender. Drain and set aside.

2 In a bowl, mix together the horseradish sauce, crème fraîche, lemon juice and oil, then season with pepper.

3 Roughly chop the apples and the warm potatoes, put in a large bowl and toss in the dressing. Skin and flake the mackerel and add to the bowl with the watercress. Toss together and serve.

Try Something Different

Try baby leaf spinach instead of watercress.
Use wholegrain Dijon mustard instead of horseradish.

EASY		NUTRITIONAL INFORMATION		Serves
Preparation Time 15 minutes	**Cooking Time** 20 minutes	**Per Serving** 320 calories, 23g fat (of which 5g saturates), 22g carbohydrate, 0.7g salt	Gluten free Dairy free	**4**

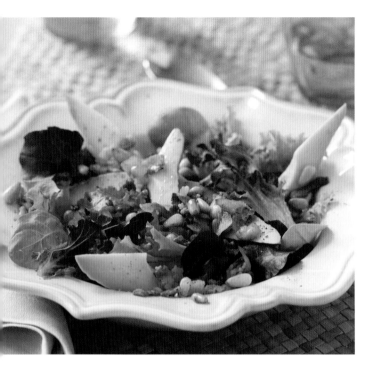

Try Something Different

Replace the pinenuts with walnuts.

Bacon, Avocado and Pinenut Salad

125g (4oz) streaky bacon rashers, de-rinded and cut into small, neat pieces (lardons)

1 shallot, finely chopped

120g bag mixed baby salad leaves

1 ripe avocado

50g (2oz) pinenuts

4 tbsp olive oil

4 tbsp red wine vinegar

salt and ground black pepper

1 Put the bacon lardons into a frying pan over a medium heat for 1–2 minutes until the fat starts to run. Add the chopped shallot and fry gently for about 5 minutes until golden.

2 Meanwhile, divide the salad leaves among four serving plates. Halve and stone the avocado, then peel, and slice the flesh. Arrange on the salad leaves.

3 Add the pinenuts, oil and wine vinegar to the frying pan and let bubble for 1 minute. Season with salt and pepper.

4 Tip the bacon, pinenuts and dressing over the salad and serve at once, while still warm.

Serves 4	EASY		NUTRITIONAL INFORMATION	
	Preparation Time 5 minutes	**Cooking Time** 7 minutes	**Per Serving** 352 calories, 34g fat (of which 6g saturates), 3g carbohydrate, 1g salt	Gluten free Dairy free

▶ Celery Soup (see page 44)
▽ Warm Chicken Liver Salad
▶ Roasted Apples with Oats and Blueberries
   (see page 119)

450g (1lb) chicken livers

1–2 tbsp balsamic vinegar

1 tsp Dijon mustard

3 tbsp olive oil

50g (2oz) streaky bacon rashers, de-rinded and cut into small, neat pieces (lardons)

50g (2oz) sun-dried tomatoes or roasted red peppers, cut into thin strips

$\frac{1}{2}$ curly endive, about 175g (6oz)

100g (3$\frac{1}{2}$oz) rocket

1 bunch spring onions, sliced

salt and ground black pepper

Warm Chicken Liver Salad

1 Drain the chicken livers on kitchen paper, then trim and cut into pieces.

2 To make the dressing, put the balsamic vinegar, mustard, 2 tbsp oil, and salt and pepper into a small bowl. Whisk together and set aside.

3 In a non-stick frying pan, fry the lardons until beginning to brown, stirring from time to time. Add the tomatoes or red pepper and heat through for 1 minute. Add the remaining oil and the chicken livers and stir-fry over a high heat for 2–3 minutes until just pink in the centre.

4 Meanwhile, toss the endive, rocket and spring onions with the dressing in a large bowl. Divide among four plates. Arrange the warm livers and bacon on top. Serve at once.

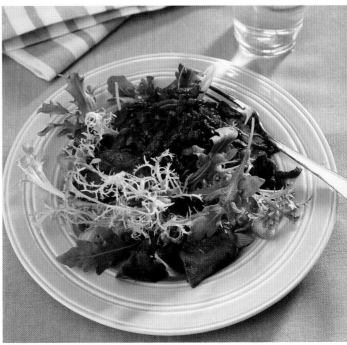

EASY		NUTRITIONAL INFORMATION		Serves
Preparation Time 20 minutes	**Cooking Time** 8–10 minutes	**Per Serving** 236 calories, 15g fat (of which 3g saturates), 3g carbohydrate, 0.8g salt	Gluten free Dairy free	**4**

Try Something Different

Instead of sardines use a 200g can salmon in oil.

Sardines on Toast

4 slices thick wholemeal bread

2 large tomatoes, sliced

2 x 120g cans sardines in olive oil, drained

juice of 1/2 lemon

small handful of parsley, chopped

1 Preheat the grill. Toast the slices of bread on both sides.

2 Divide the tomato slices and the sardines among the toast slices, squeeze the lemon juice over them, then put back under the grill for 2–3 minutes to heat through. Scatter the parsley over the sardines and serve immediately.

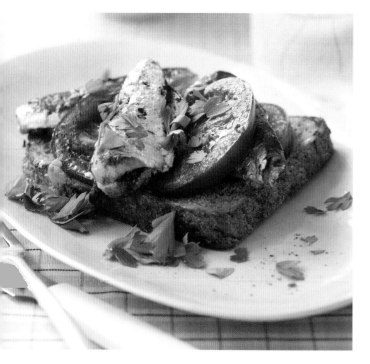

Serves 4	**EASY**		**NUTRITIONAL INFORMATION**	
	Preparation Time 5 minutes	Cooking Time 8–10 minutes	Per Serving 240 calories, 9g fat (of which 2g saturates), 25g carbohydrate, 1.6g salt	Gluten free Dairy free

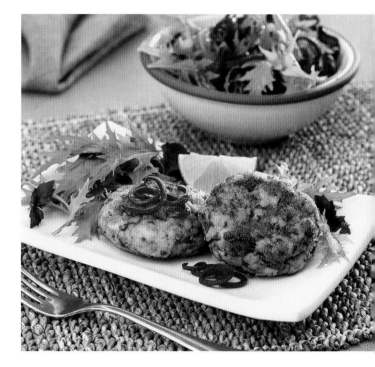

Quick Crab Cakes

200g (7oz) fresh crabmeat

2 spring onions, finely chopped

2 red chillies, seeded and finely chopped (see page 71)

finely grated zest of 1 lime

4 tbsp freshly chopped coriander

about 40g (1½oz) stoneground wholemeal breadcrumbs

1 tbsp groundnut oil

1 tbsp plain flour

thinly sliced red chilli to garnish

1 lime, cut into wedges, and salad leaves to serve

1   Put the crabmeat in a bowl, then mix with the spring onions, chillies, lime zest and coriander. Add enough breadcrumbs to hold the mixture together, then form into four small patties.

2   Heat ½ tbsp oil in a pan. Dredge the patties with flour and fry on one side for 3 minutes. Add the rest of the oil, turn the patties over and fry for a further 2–3 minutes. Garnish the crab cakes with thinly sliced red chilli and serve with lime wedges to squeeze over them, and salad leaves.

EASY		NUTRITIONAL INFORMATION		Serves
Preparation Time 15 minutes	**Cooking Time** 6 minutes	**Per Serving** 124 calories, 4g fat (of which 1g saturates), 12g carbohydrate, 0.9g salt	Gluten free Dairy free	**4**

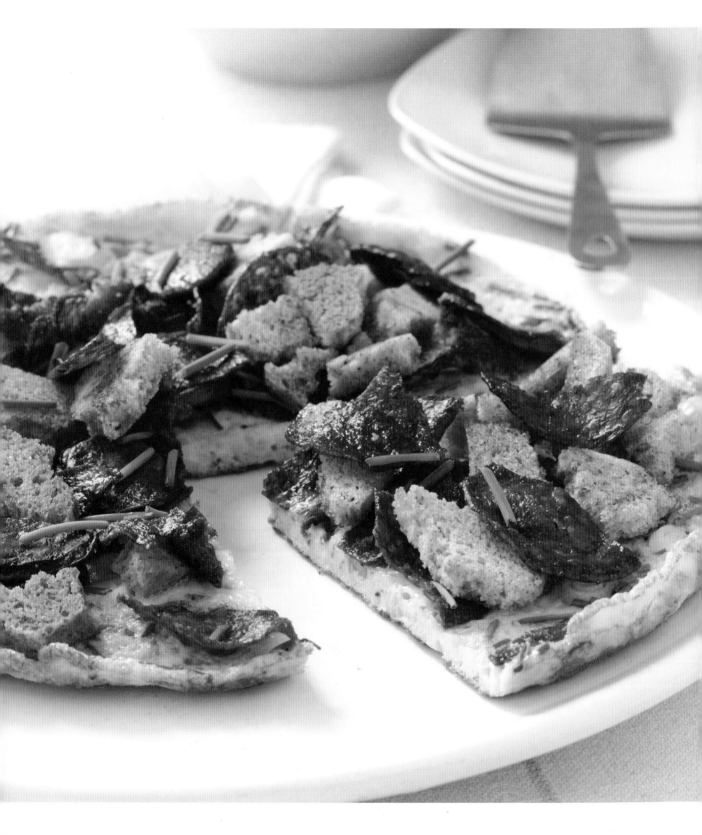

Spanish Omelette

225g (8oz) piece salami, chorizo or garlic sausage, sliced or roughly chopped

50g (2oz) slightly stale sourdough bread (crusts removed), roughly chopped

8 large eggs

2 spring onions, finely chopped

1 small bunch chives, finely chopped, plus extra to garnish

ground black pepper

green salad to serve

1 Heat a large, 28cm (11in), heavy-based frying pan, add the sausage pieces and fry over a low heat until the fat begins to run. Increase the heat and cook the sausage until golden and crisp. Remove from the pan (leaving the fat in the pan) and set aside. Add the bread to the pan and fry until it's also golden and crisp. Remove the pan from the heat, mix the croûtons with the cooked sausage and keep warm.

2 In a bowl, beat together the eggs, spring onions and chives, then season with pepper. Heat the pan used for the salami and bread. When very hot, add the egg mixture, allowing the liquid to spread across the base of the pan. Cook for 2 minutes, then, using a spatula, draw the cooked edges into the centre, tilting the pan so the mixture runs into the gaps.

3 When the omelette is almost set, reduce the heat and spoon the salami and croûton mixture evenly over the top. Cook for a further 30 seconds, then cut the omelette into four wedges. Sprinkle with chives and serve with a green salad.

EASY		NUTRITIONAL INFORMATION		Serves
Preparation Time 5 minutes	**Cooking Time** 15 minutes	**Per Serving** 466 calories, 36g fat (of which 12g saturates), 7g carbohydrate, 3.1g salt	Gluten free Dairy free	**4**

Try Something Different

Try quinoa (see page 18) instead of the bulgur wheat.

Beef Tomatoes with Bulgur

125g (4oz) bulgur wheat

20g (³⁄₄oz) flat-leafed parsley, finely chopped

75g (3oz) feta cheese, chopped

1 courgette, chopped

50g (2oz) flaked almonds, toasted

4 large beef tomatoes

1 tbsp olive oil

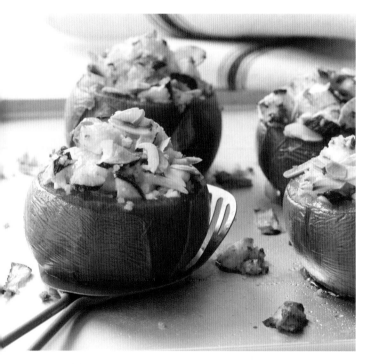

1 Preheat the oven to 180°C (160°C fan oven) mark 4. Cook the bulgur according to the packet instructions. Chop the parsley, feta and courgette and stir into the bulgur with the almonds.

2 Chop the top off each tomato and scoop out the seeds. Put on to a baking sheet and spoon in the bulgur mixture. Drizzle with the oil and cook in the oven for 15–20 minutes until the cheese is starting to soften.

Serves 4	EASY		NUTRITIONAL INFORMATION	
	Preparation Time 10 minutes	**Cooking Time** 30–35 minutes	**Per Serving** 245 calories, 14g fat (of which 4g saturates), 21g carbohydrate, 0.7g salt	Vegetarian

Try Something Different

Diced ripe avocado can be added. It is rich in omega fats and is good for your skin.

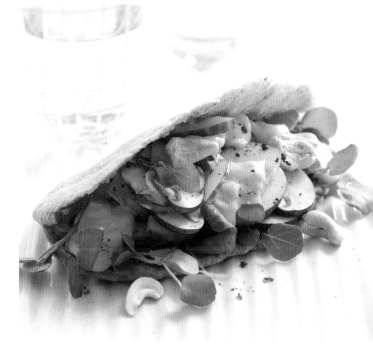

Veggie Pitta

1 wholemeal pitta bread
1 tbsp hummus (see page 66), plus extra to serve
15g (¹/₂oz) unsalted cashew nuts
2 closed cup mushrooms, finely sliced
¹/₄ cucumber, chopped
fresh watercress or mixed salad leaves
ground black pepper

1 Split the pitta bread and spread with the hummus.

2 Fill the pitta with the cashew nuts, mushrooms, cucumber and a generous helping of fresh watercress or mixed salad leaves. Serve with extra hummus if you like, and season with pepper.

EASY	NUTRITIONAL INFORMATION		Serves
Preparation Time 8 minutes	**Per Serving** 322 calories, 11g fat (of which 2g saturates), 47g carbohydrate, 1.2g salt	Vegetarian	**1**

Lemon Hummus with Black Olives

2 x 400g cans chickpeas, drained and rinsed

1 garlic clove (use fresh garlic when possible, see Cook's Tips), crushed

zest and juice of 1 lemon

4 tbsp olive oil

25g (1oz) pitted black olives, roughly chopped

1 tsp paprika, plus a little extra

sticks of raw vegetables and breadsticks to serve

1 Put the chickpeas and garlic into a food processor with the chickpeas. Add the lemon zest and juice and whiz to combine. With the motor running, drizzle in the oil to make a thick paste. If the hummus is too thick, add 1–2 tbsp cold water and whiz again.

2 Spoon into a bowl and stir in the olives and paprika. Serve with a sprinkling of extra paprika, if you like, with raw vegetables and breadsticks for dipping.

Cook's Tips

Raw garlic is renowned for its curative and protective powers, which include lowering blood pressure and cholesterol levels.

Fresh garlic has juicy, mild cloves and is available from May throughout the summer. It is the classic form of garlic to use for making, for example, pesto, salsa verde, garlic mayonnaise and chilled soups.

Serves 4	EASY	NUTRITIONAL INFORMATION	
	Preparation Time 15 minutes	**Per Serving** 284 calories, 16g fat (of which 2g saturates), 25g carbohydrate, 1.2g salt	Vegetarian Gluten free • Dairy free

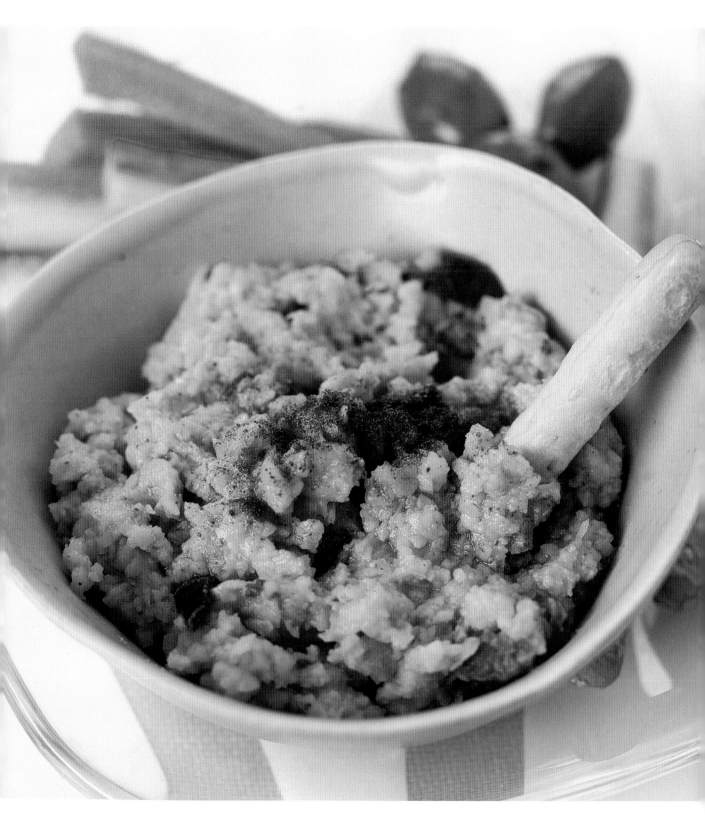

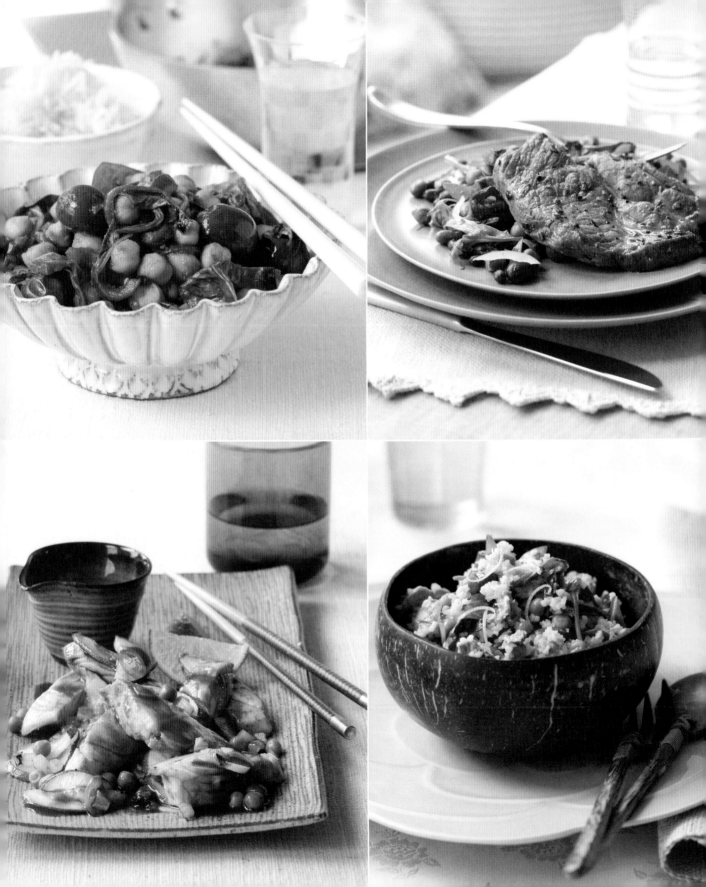

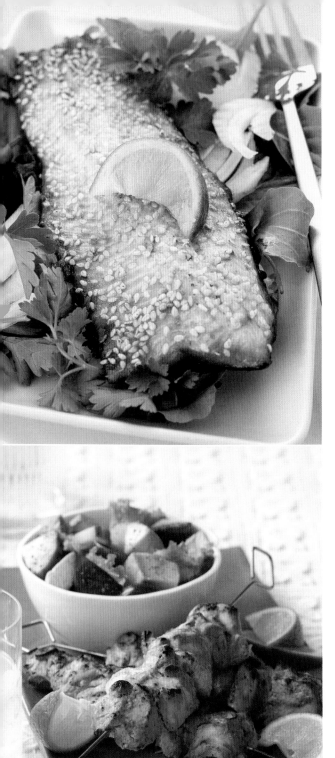

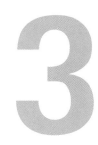

3

Easy Suppers

Try Something Different

Use pork fillet instead of turkey, cutting the fillet across into thin slices.

2 tbsp vegetable or sunflower oil

500g (1lb 2oz) turkey fillet, cut into strips

2 garlic cloves, crushed

2.5cm (1in) piece fresh root ginger, grated

1 broccoli head, chopped into florets

8 spring onions, finely chopped

125g (4oz) button mushrooms, halved

100g (3½oz) bean sprouts

3 tbsp oyster sauce

1 tbsp light soy sauce

125ml (4fl oz) hot chicken stock

juice of ½ lemon

egg noodles to serve

Turkey and Broccoli Stir-fry

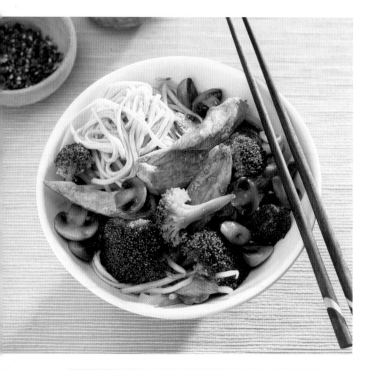

1 Heat 1 tbsp oil in a large, non-stick frying pan or wok, add the turkey strips and stir-fry for 4–5 minutes until golden and cooked through. Remove from the pan and set aside.

2 Heat the remaining oil in the same pan over a medium heat, add the garlic and ginger and cook for 30 seconds, stirring all the time so they don't burn. Add the broccoli, spring onions and mushrooms, turn up the heat and cook for 2–3 minutes until the vegetables start to brown but are still crisp.

3 Return the turkey to the pan and add the bean sprouts, sauces, stock and lemon juice. Cook for 1–2 minutes, tossing well to heat everything through, then serve with egg noodles.

Serves 4	EASY		NUTRITIONAL INFORMATION	
	Preparation Time 15 minutes	**Cooking Time** 8–12 minutes	**Per Serving** 250 calories, 8g fat (of which 1g saturates), 7g carbohydrate, 1.2g salt	Gluten free Dairy free

Cook's Tip

Chillies vary enormously in strength, from quite mild to blisteringly hot, depending on the type of chilli and its ripeness. Taste a small piece first to check it's not too hot for you.

Be extremely careful when handling chillies not to touch or rub your eyes with your fingers, as they will sting. Wash knives immediately after handling chillies for the same reason. As a precaution, use rubber gloves when preparing them if you like.

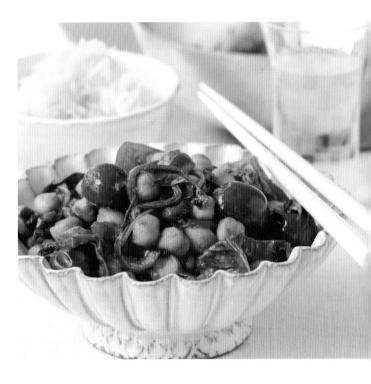

Chickpea and Chilli Stir-fry

2 tbsp olive oil

1 tsp ground cumin

1 red onion, sliced

2 garlic cloves, finely chopped

1 red chilli, seeded and finely chopped (see Cook's Tip)

2 x 400g cans chickpeas, rinsed and drained

400g (14oz) cherry tomatoes

125g (4oz) baby spinach leaves

brown rice or pasta to serve

1 Heat the oil in a wok. Add the ground cumin and fry for 1–2 minutes. Add the onion and stir-fry for 5–7 minutes.

2 Add the garlic and chilli and stir-fry for 2 minutes.

3 Add the chickpeas to the wok with the tomatoes. Reduce the heat and simmer until the chickpeas are hot. Add the spinach and stir to wilt. Serve with brown rice or pasta.

EASY		NUTRITIONAL INFORMATION		Serves
Preparation Time 10 minutes	**Cooking Time** 15–20 minutes	**Per Serving** 258 calories, 11g fat (of which 1g saturates), 30g carbohydrate, 1g salt	Vegetarian Gluten free • Dairy free	**4**

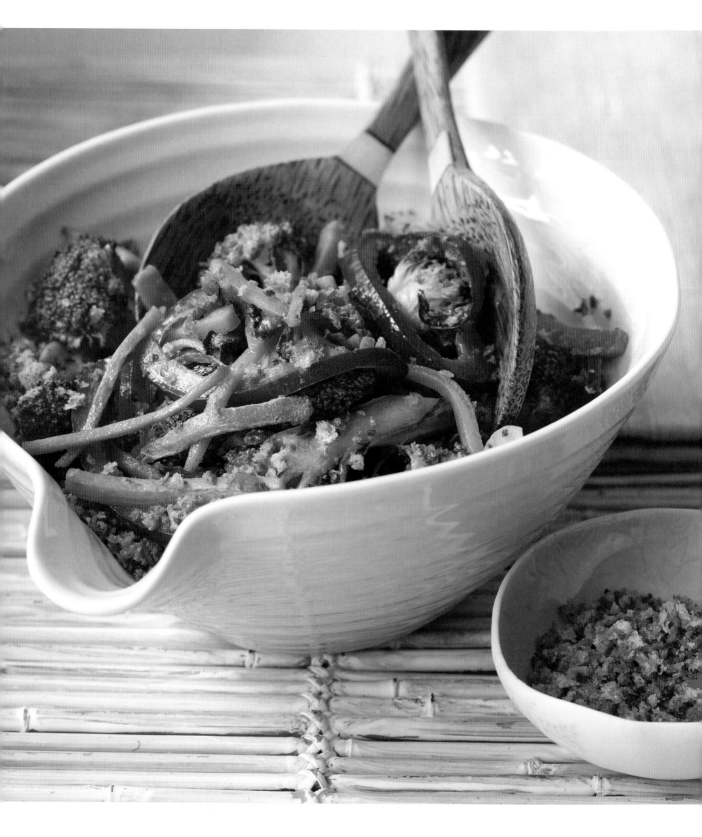

Stir-fried Veg with Crispy Crumbs

1 thick slice wholemeal bread, crusts removed

2 tbsp olive oil

1 broccoli head, chopped into florets

1 large carrot, cut into thin strips

1 red pepper, cut into thin strips

4 anchovy fillets, chopped

1 Whiz the bread in a food processor to make breadcrumbs. Heat 1 tbsp oil in a large, non-stick frying pan or wok. Add the breadcrumbs and stir-fry for 4–5 minutes until crisp. Remove from the pan and set aside on a piece of kitchen paper.

2 Heat the remaining oil in the frying pan until hot. Add the broccoli, carrot and pepper and stir-fry over a high heat for 4–5 minutes until they're starting to soften. Add the anchovies and continue to cook for a further 5 minutes until slightly softened. Serve the vegetables immediately, scattered with the breadcrumbs.

Try Something Different

Use other vegetables in season: try 400g (14oz) cauliflower florets instead of the broccoli.

EASY		NUTRITIONAL INFORMATION		Serves
Preparation Time 10 minutes	**Cooking Time** 15–20 minutes	**Per Serving** 145 calories, 8g fat (of which 1g saturates), 13g carbohydrate, 0.5g salt	Dairy free	**4**

▶ Winter Leaf Salad (see page 50)
▼ Tomato and Artichoke Pasta
▶ Rhubarb and Raspberry Meringue
  (see page 113)

Tomato and Artichoke Pasta

300g (11oz) penne

6 pieces sunblush tomatoes in oil

1 red onion, sliced

about 10 pieces roasted artichoke hearts in oil, drained and roughly chopped

50g (2oz) pitted black olives, roughly chopped

50g (2oz) pecorino cheese, grated

100g (3½oz) rocket

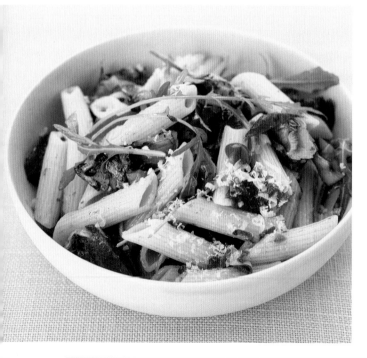

1 Cook the pasta in a large pan of boiling water according to the packet instructions; do not overcook – it should be al dente. Drain well.

2 Meanwhile, drain the sunblush tomatoes, reserving the oil, and roughly chop. Heat 1 tbsp oil from the tomatoes in a large frying pan, add the onion and fry for 5–6 minutes until softened and turning golden. Add the tomatoes, artichokes and olives to the pan and heat for 3–4 minutes until hot.

3 Add half the pecorino cheese and stir through. Remove from the heat and stir in the rocket and pasta. Divide the pasta among four bowls and sprinkle the remaining pecorino over the top to serve.

Serves 4	EASY		NUTRITIONAL INFORMATION	
	Preparation Time 10 minutes	**Cooking Time** 10–12 minutes	**Per Serving** 380 calories, 11g fat (of which 4g saturates), 59g carbohydrate, 1.3g salt	Vegetarian

Try Something Different

Use rocket instead of spinach – no need to chop.

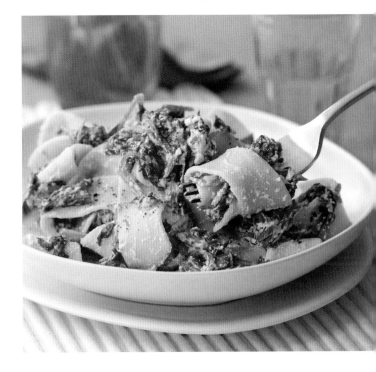

Pappardelle with Spinach

350g (12oz) pappardelle

350g (12oz) baby leaf spinach, roughly chopped

2 tbsp olive oil

75g (3oz) ricotta

freshly grated nutmeg

salt and ground black pepper

1　Cook the pappardelle in a large pan of boiling water according to the packet instructions.

2　Drain the pasta well, return to the pan and add the spinach, oil and ricotta, tossing for 10–15 seconds or until the spinach has wilted. Season with a little freshly grated nutmeg and salt and pepper and serve immediately.

EASY		NUTRITIONAL INFORMATION		Serves
Preparation Time 10 minutes	**Cooking Time** 12 minutes	**Per Serving** 404 calories, 11g fat (of which 3g saturates), 67g carbohydrate, 0.3g salt	Vegetarian	**4**

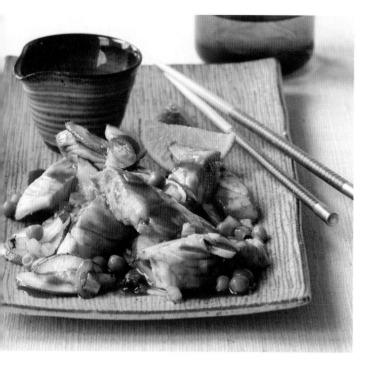

Try Something Different

There are plenty of alternatives to haddock: try sea bass, sea bream or gurnard.

Chinese-style Fish

2 tsp sunflower oil

1 small onion, finely chopped

1 green chilli, seeded and finely chopped (see page 71)

2 courgettes, thinly sliced

125g (4oz) frozen peas (defrosted)

350g (12oz) skinless haddock fillet, cut into bite-sized pieces

2 tsp lemon juice

4 tbsp hoisin sauce

lime wedges to serve

1 Heat the oil in a large, non-stick frying pan. Add the onion, chilli, courgettes and peas. Stir over a high heat for 5 minutes until the onion and courgettes begin to soften.

2 Add the fish to the pan with the lemon juice, hoisin sauce and 150ml (¼ pint) water. Bring to the boil, then simmer, uncovered, for 2–3 minutes until the fish is cooked through. Serve with lime wedges.

Serves 4	EASY		NUTRITIONAL INFORMATION	
	Preparation Time 5 minutes	**Cooking Time** 10 minutes	**Per Serving** 150 calories, 3g fat (of which 1g saturates), 10g carbohydrate, 0.7g salt	Gluten free Dairy free

Cook's Tip

Sesame seeds are deliciously nutty and highly nutritious. They are a valuable source of protein, good omega fats and vitamin E. Lightly toasted sesame seeds, crushed with a little salt and stirred into 1–2 tbsp of olive oil, make an excellent dressing for cooked green beans, broccoli and carrots.

Crusted Trout

1 tbsp sesame oil

1 tbsp soy sauce

juice of 1 lime

4 x 150g (5oz) trout fillets

2 tbsp sesame seeds

lime wedges, herb salad and fennel to serve

1 Preheat the grill. Put the sesame oil in a bowl. Add the soy sauce and lime juice and whisk together.

2 Put the trout fillets on a baking sheet, pour the sesame mixture over them and grill for 8–10 minutes. Sprinkle with the sesame seeds and grill for a further 2–3 minutes until the seeds are golden. Serve with lime wedges, a herb salad and some finely sliced fennel.

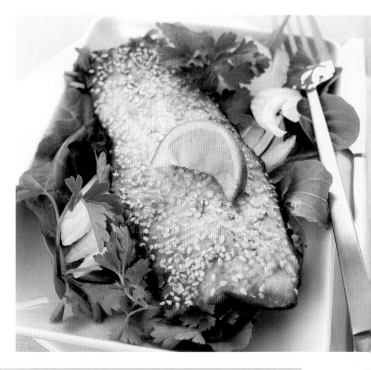

EASY		NUTRITIONAL INFORMATION		Serves
Preparation Time 10 minutes	**Cooking Time** 10–13 minutes	**Per Serving** 259 calories, 15g fat (of which 3g saturates), 1g carbohydrate, 0.8g salt	Gluten free Dairy free	4

Prawn, Courgette and Leek Risotto

1 tbsp olive oil
25g (1oz) butter
1 leek, finely chopped
2 courgettes, finely chopped
2 garlic cloves, crushed
350g (12oz) arborio (risotto) rice
100ml (3½fl oz) dry white wine
1.6 litres (2¾ pints) hot vegetable stock
200g (7oz) cooked prawns
small bunch parsley or mint, or a mixture of both
salt and ground black pepper
green salad or green beans to serve

1 In a large, shallow pan, heat the oil and half the butter, then add the leek, courgettes and garlic and soften over a low heat. Add the rice and stir well, so it soaks up the melted butter, and cook for 1 minute, then pour in the wine. Let bubble until the wine has evaporated.

2 Meanwhile, in another large pan, heat the stock to a low, steady simmer. Ladle the stock into the risotto gradually, adding the next ladleful only when all the stock has been absorbed. Stir constantly to ensure that the risotto is creamy.

3 When nearly all the stock has been added and the rice is al dente (just tender but with a little bite at the centre), add the cooked prawns. Season to taste and stir in the remaining stock and the rest of the butter. Stir through and take off the heat. Cover and leave to stand for a couple of minutes, then stir the chopped herbs through.

4 Serve immediately with a green salad or cooked green beans.

Serves 6	EASY		NUTRITIONAL INFORMATION	
	Preparation Time 10 minutes	Cooking Time 30 minutes	Per Serving 320 calories, 7g fat (of which 3g saturates), 49g carbohydrate, 1.3g salt	Gluten free Dairy free

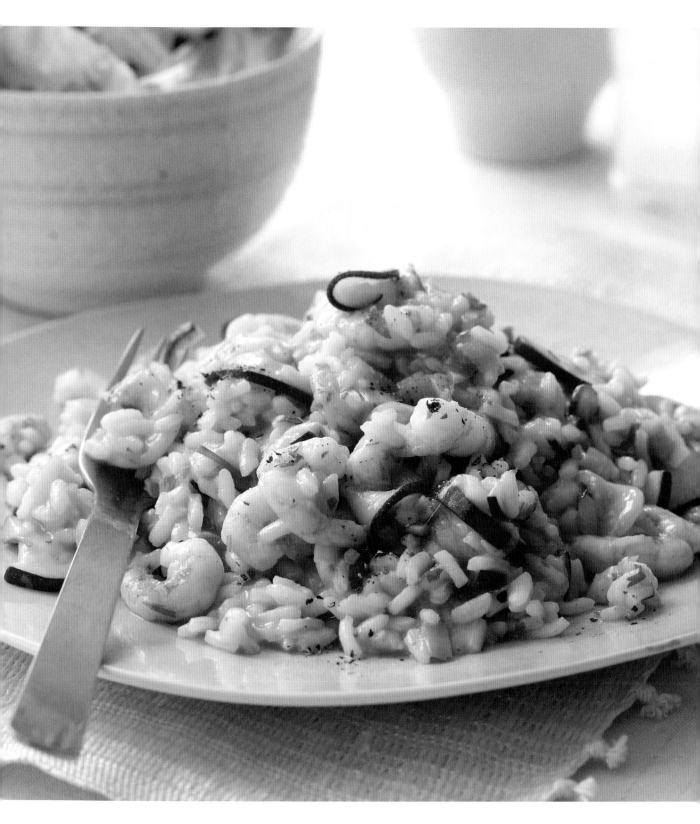

Tomato Risotto

1 large rosemary sprig

2 tbsp olive oil

1 small onion, finely chopped

300g (11oz) cherry tomatoes, halved

350g (12oz) risotto (arborio) rice

4 tbsp dry white wine

750ml (1¼ pints) hot vegetable stock

salt and ground black pepper

shavings of Parmesan, green salad and extra virgin olive oil to serve

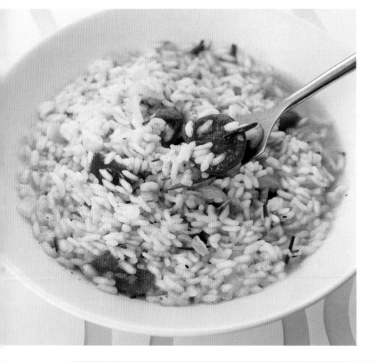

1 Pull the leaves from the rosemary and chop roughly. Set aside.

2 Heat the oil in a flameproof casserole, add the onion and cook for about 8–10 minutes until beginning to soften. Add the rice and stir to coat in the oil and onion. Pour in the wine, then the hot stock, stirring well to mix.

3 Bring to the boil, stirring, then cover and simmer for 5 minutes. Stir in the tomatoes and chopped rosemary. Simmer, covered, for a further 10–15 minutes or until the rice is tender and most of the liquid has been absorbed. Season to taste.

4 Serve immediately with shavings of Parmesan, a large green salad and extra virgin olive oil to drizzle over.

Serves 6	EASY		NUTRITIONAL INFORMATION	
	Preparation Time 10 minutes	**Cooking Time** 25–30 minutes	**Per Serving** 264 calories, 4g fat (of which 1g saturates), 49g carbohydrate, 0.5g salt	Vegetarian Gluten free

Try Something Different

Instead of salmon use 200g (7oz) cooked peeled prawns and 200g (7oz) cherry tomatoes.

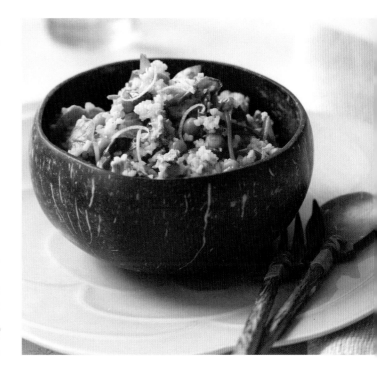

Salmon and Bulgur Wheat Pilaf

1 tbsp olive oil

1 onion, chopped

175g (6oz) bulgur wheat

450ml (¾ pint) vegetable stock

400g can pink salmon, drained and flaked

125g (4oz) spinach, roughly chopped

225g (8oz) frozen peas

zest and juice of 1 lemon

salt and ground black pepper

1 Heat the oil in a large saucepan, add the onion and cook until softened. Stir in the bulgur wheat to coat in the oil, then stir in the stock and bring to the boil. Cover, reduce the heat and simmer for 10–15 minutes until the stock has been fully absorbed.

2 Stir in the salmon, spinach, peas and lemon juice and cook until the spinach has wilted and the salmon and peas are heated through. Season and sprinkle with lemon zest before serving.

EASY		NUTRITIONAL INFORMATION		Serves
Preparation Time 5 minutes	**Cooking Time** 20 minutes	**Per Serving** 323 calories, 11g fat (of which 2g saturates), 30g carbohydrate, 1.5g salt	Dairy free	**4**

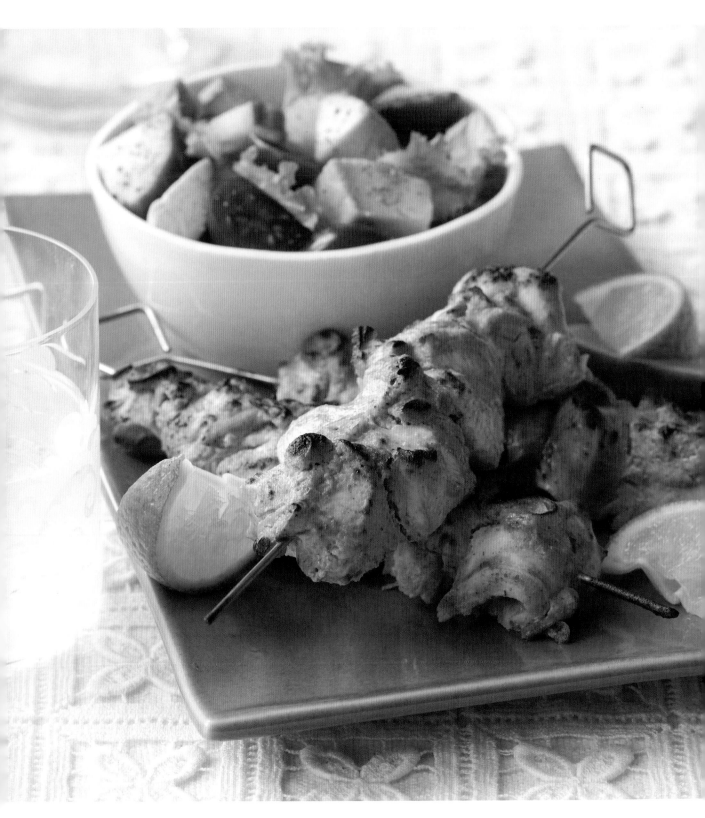

Spiced Tikka Kebabs

2 tbsp tikka paste

150g (5oz) natural yogurt

juice of $\frac{1}{2}$ lime

4 spring onions, chopped

350g (12oz) skinless chicken, cut into bite-sized pieces

lime wedges to serve

1 Preheat the grill. Put the tikka paste, yogurt, lime juice and chopped spring onions into a large bowl. Add the chicken and toss well. Thread the chicken on to skewers.

2 Grill for 8–10 minutes on each side or until cooked through, turning and basting with the paste. Serve with lime wedges to squeeze over the kebabs.

Cook's Tip

Serve with rocket salad: put 75g (3oz) rocket in a large bowl. Add $\frac{1}{4}$ chopped avocado, a handful of halved cherry tomatoes, $\frac{1}{2}$ chopped cucumber and the juice of 1 lime. Season with salt and pepper and mix together.

EASY		NUTRITIONAL INFORMATION		Serves
Preparation Time 10 minutes	**Cooking Time** 20 minutes	**Per Serving** 150 calories, 5g fat (of which 1g saturates), 4g carbohydrate, 0.3g salt	Gluten free	**4**

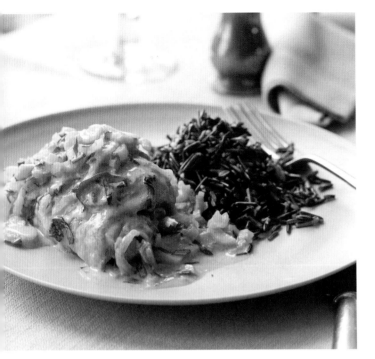

Chicken with Fennel and Tarragon

1 tbsp olive oil
4 chicken thighs
1 onion, finely chopped
1 fennel bulb, sliced
juice of ½ lemon
200ml (7fl oz) hot chicken stock
200g (7oz) half-fat crème fraîche
1 small bunch tarragon, roughly chopped
wild rice to serve

1 Preheat the oven to 200°C (180°C fan) mark 6. Heat the olive oil in a large flameproof casserole. Add the chicken thighs and fry for 5 minutes until brown, then remove and set them aside to keep warm.

2 Add the onion to the pan and fry for 5 minutes, then add the fennel and cook for 5–10 minutes until softened.

3 Add the lemon juice to the pan, then add the stock. Bring to a simmer and cook until the liquid is reduced by half.

4 Stir in the crème fraîche and return the chicken to the pan. Stir once to mix, then cover and cook in the oven for 25–30 minutes. Stir the tarragon into the sauce and serve with wild rice.

Serves 4	EASY		NUTRITIONAL INFORMATION	
	Preparation Time 10 minutes	Cooking Time 45–55 minutes	Per Serving 334 calories, 26g fat (of which 15g saturates), 3g carbohydrate, 0.5g salt	Gluten free

2 tbsp each soy sauce and Worcestershire sauce

2 tsp tomato purée

juice of $\frac{1}{2}$ lemon

1 tbsp sesame seeds

1 garlic clove, crushed

400g (14oz) rump steak, sliced

1 tbsp vegetable oil

3 small pak choi, chopped

1 bunch spring onions, sliced

egg noodles to serve

Sesame Beef

1 In a bowl, mix together the soy and Worcestershire sauces, tomato purée, lemon juice, sesame seeds and garlic. Add the steak and toss to coat.

2 Heat the oil in a large wok or non-stick frying pan until hot. Add the steak and sear well. Remove from the wok and set aside.

3 Add any sauce from the bowl to the wok and heat for 1 minute. Add the pak choi, spring onions and steak, and stir-fry for 5 minutes. Serve immediately, with egg noodles.

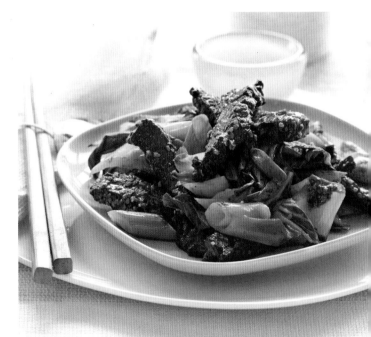

EASY		NUTRITIONAL INFORMATION		Serves
Preparation Time 20 minutes	**Cooking Time** 10 minutes	**Per Serving** 207 calories, 10g fat (of which 3g saturates), 4g carbohydrate, 2g salt	Dairy free	**4**

Cook's Tip

Serve with chilli coleslaw: put 3 peeled and finely shredded carrots in a large bowl. Add $^1/_2$ finely shredded white cabbage, 1 finely sliced, seeded red pepper and $^1/_2$ chopped cucumber. In a small bowl, mix together $^1/_2$ tsp harissa, 100g (3$^1/_2$oz) natural yogurt and 1 tbsp white wine vinegar. Add to the vegetables and toss well.

Healthy Burgers

450g (1lb) top-quality lean minced beef

1 onion, very finely chopped

1 tbsp dried herbes de Provence

2 tsp sun-dried tomato paste

1 medium egg, beaten

ground black pepper

1 In a bowl, mix together the minced beef, onion, herbs, sun-dried tomato paste and beaten egg. Season with pepper, then shape the mixture into four round burgers about 2cm ($^3/_4$in) thick.

2 Preheat the grill or griddle pan. Cook the burgers for 4–6 minutes on each side.

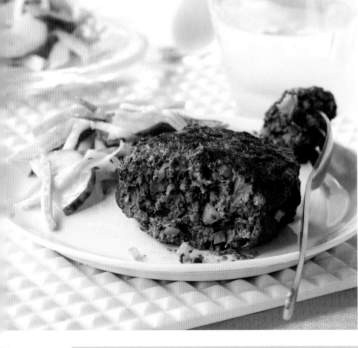

Serves 4	EASY		NUTRITIONAL INFORMATION	
	Preparation Time 10 minutes	**Cooking Time** 8–12 minutes	**Per Serving** 80 calories, 20g fat (of which 8g saturates), 2g carbohydrate, 0.3g salt	Gluten free Dairy free

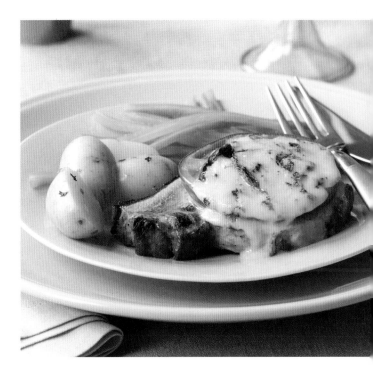

Pork with Basil, Tomato and Stilton

4 pork loin steaks
1 ripe beef tomato, sliced
few basil leaves
50g (2oz) Stilton cheese, sliced
new potatoes and runner beans to serve

1 Preheat the grill. Grill the pork for 4–5 minutes on each side.

2 Divide the sliced tomato among the steaks, with a few basil leaves and the sliced Stilton, and grill for a further 1–2 minutes until the cheese has melted and the pork is cooked through. Serve with new potatoes and runner beans.

Try Something Different

Instead of pork use 4 skinless boneless chicken breasts: season lightly, place between two pieces of clingfilm and beat with a rolling pin until about 1cm (½in) thick. Brush lightly with olive oil before grilling.

EASY		NUTRITIONAL INFORMATION		Serves
Preparation Time 10 minutes	**Cooking Time** 10–14 minutes	**Per Serving** 212 calories, 9g fat (of which 5g saturates), 2g carbohydrate, 0.5g salt	Gluten free	**4**

Lamb Steaks with Mixed Bean Salad

150g (5oz) sunblush tomatoes in oil
1 garlic clove, crushed
2 rosemary sprigs
4 x 175g (6oz) leg of lamb steaks
$\frac{1}{2}$ small red onion, finely sliced
2 x 400g cans mixed beans, drained and rinsed
large handful of rocket
salt and ground black pepper

1 Preheat the grill to high. Drain the sunblush tomatoes, reserving the oil. Put the garlic in a large, shallow dish with 1 tbsp oil from the tomatoes. Strip the leaves from the rosemary sprigs, snip into small pieces and add to the dish. Season with salt and pepper, then add the lamb and toss to coat.

2 Grill the lamb for 3–4 minutes on each side until cooked but still just pink. Meanwhile, roughly chop the tomatoes and put into a pan with the onion, beans, remaining rosemary, rocket and a further 1 tbsp oil from the tomatoes. Warm through until the rocket starts to wilt. Serve the lamb steaks with the bean salad on warmed plates.

▶ Bacon, Avocado and Pinenut Salad (see page 58)
▲ Lamb Steaks with Mixed Bean Salad
▶ Poached Peaches and Strawberries (see page 117)

Serves 4	EASY		NUTRITIONAL INFORMATION	
	Preparation Time 5 minutes	**Cooking Time** 10 minutes	**Per Serving** 545 calories, 20g fat (of which 7g saturates), 30g carbohydrate, 1.8g salt	Gluten free Dairy free

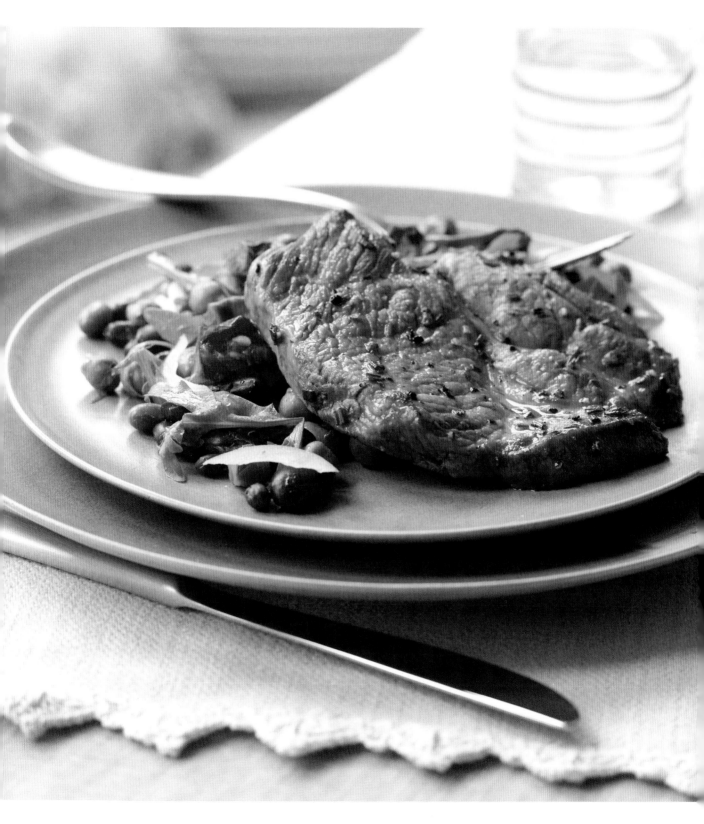

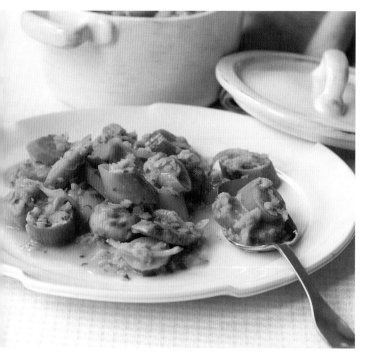

Lentil Casserole

2 tbsp olive oil

2 onions, sliced

4 carrots, sliced

3 leeks, sliced

450g (1lb) button mushrooms

2 garlic cloves, crushed

2.5cm (1in) piece fresh root ginger, grated

1 tbsp ground coriander

225g (8oz) split red lentils

750ml (1¼ pints) hot vegetable stock

4 tbsp freshly chopped coriander

salt and ground black pepper

1 Preheat the oven to 180°C (160°C fan oven) mark 4. Heat the oil in a flameproof, ovenproof casserole, add the onions, carrots and leeks and fry, stirring, for 5 minutes. Add the mushrooms, garlic, ginger and ground coriander, and fry for 2–3 minutes.

2 Rinse and drain the lentils, then stir into the casserole with the stock. Season with salt and pepper and return to the boil. Cover and cook in the oven for 45–50 minutes until the vegetables and lentils are tender. Stir in the chopped coriander before serving.

Serves 6	EASY		NUTRITIONAL INFORMATION	
	Preparation Time 20 minutes	**Cooking Time** 1 hour	**Per Serving** 239 calories, 6g fat (of which 1g saturates), 36g carbohydrate, 0.4g salt	Vegetarian Gluten free • Dairy free

225g (8oz) green beans

3 tbsp olive oil

2 onions, finely chopped

2 garlic cloves, finely chopped

2 small green chillies, seeded and finely chopped (see page 71)

1 tsp each ground turmeric, paprika and garam masala

1 tbsp each ground cumin and ground coriander

4 tomatoes, roughly chopped

2 tbsp freshly chopped coriander

1 tbsp freshly chopped mint

400g can chickpeas, drained and rinsed

400g can haricot beans, drained and rinsed

salt and ground black pepper

Chickpeas with Tomato and Green Beans

1 Cook the green beans in a pan of boiling water for 4–5 minutes until just tender. Drain and set aside until needed. Heat the oil in a heavy-based pan, add the onions and garlic, and fry gently for 5 minutes. Add the chillies to the pan together with the spices and cook, stirring, for a further 1–2 minutes.

2 Add the tomatoes to the pan with the chopped coriander and mint. Season with salt and pepper. Cook, stirring, for 5–10 minutes until the tomatoes are soft.

3 Add the chickpeas and haricot beans to the pan together with the reserved green beans. Simmer until the chickpeas are hot. Serve on its own or with roast chicken or lamb.

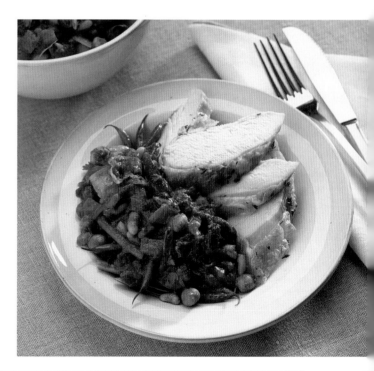

EASY		NUTRITIONAL INFORMATION		Serves
Preparation Time 10 minutes	**Cooking Time** 20–25 minutes	**Per Serving** 350 calories, 13g fat (of which 2g saturates), 45g carbohydrate, 1.2g salt	Gluten free • Dairy free	4

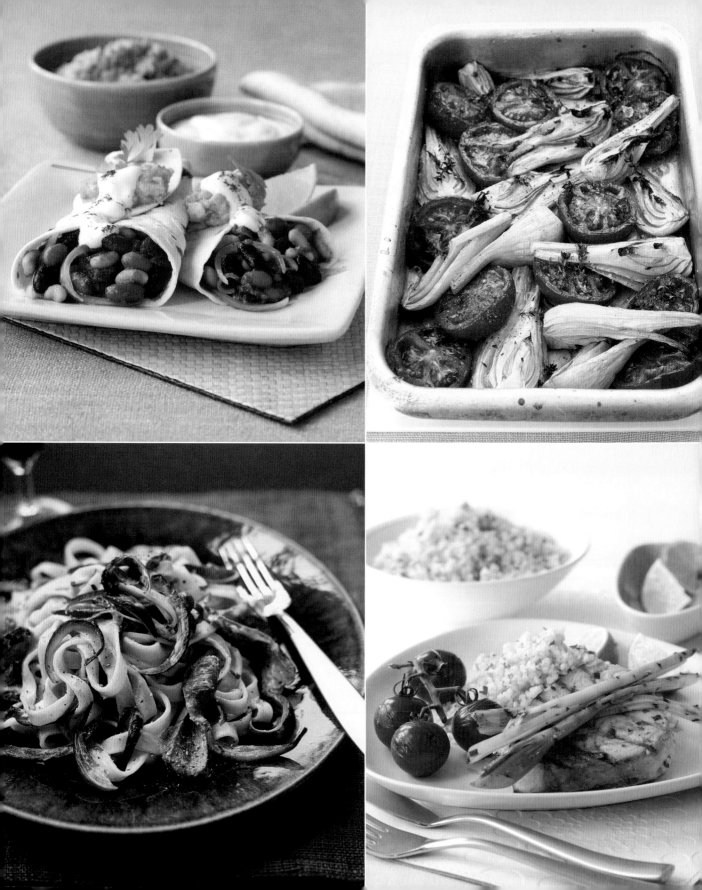

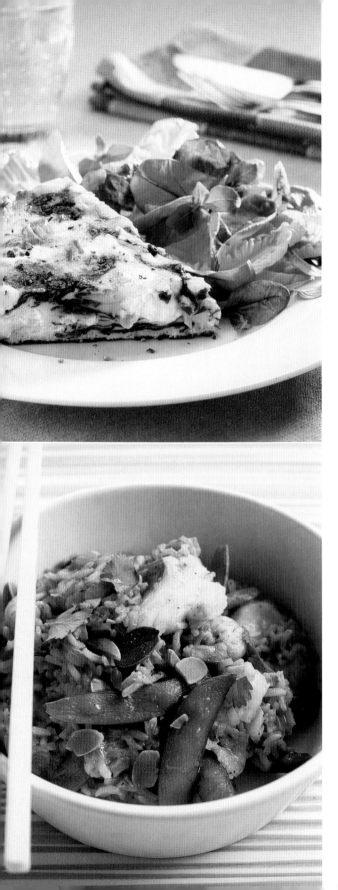

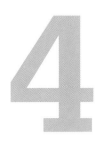

Food for Friends

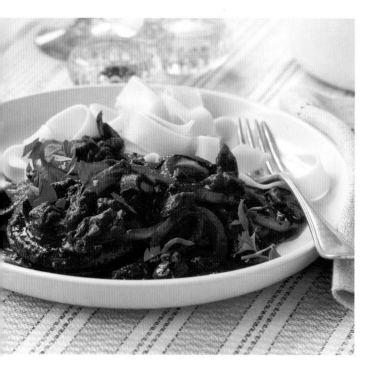

▶ Smoked Mackerel with Potato and
  Horseradish Salad (see page 57)
▼ Italian Sausage Stew
▶ Lemon Sorbet (see page 111)

Italian Sausage Stew

25g (1oz) dried porcini mushrooms
300g (11oz) whole rustic Italian salami sausages,
such as salami Milano
2 tbsp olive oil
1 onion, sliced
2 garlic cloves, chopped
1 small red chilli, seeded and chopped (see page 71)
1 rosemary sprig
400g can chopped tomatoes
200ml (7fl oz) red wine
ground black pepper
freshly chopped flat-leafed parsley to garnish
tagliatelle or fettucine to serve

1 Put the dried mushrooms in a small bowl, pour on
100ml (3½fl oz) boiling water and leave to soak for
20 minutes, or soften in the microwave on full power
for 3½ minutes and leave to cool. Cut the salami
into 1cm (½in) slices and set aside.

2 Heat the olive oil in a pan, add the onion, garlic
and chilli and fry gently for 5 minutes. Meanwhile,
strip the leaves from the rosemary sprig and add
them to the pan, stirring. Add the salami and fry for
2 minutes on each side or until browned. Drain and
chop the mushrooms and add them to the pan. Stir
in the chopped tomatoes and red wine, then season
with pepper. Simmer, uncovered, for 5 minutes.
Sprinkle with parsley and serve with tagliatelle or
fettucine.

Serves 4	EASY		NUTRITIONAL INFORMATION	
	Preparation Time 10 minutes	**Cooking Time** 15 minutes	**Per Serving** 443 calories, 35g fat (of which 12g saturates), 6g carbohydrate, 3.4g salt	Dairy free

Try Something Different

Use white wine instead of apple juice.

Pork Steaks with Sage and Parma Ham

4 pork shoulder steaks, about 150g (5oz) each

4 thin slices Parma ham or pancetta

6 sage leaves

1 tbsp oil

150ml (¼ pint) pure unsweetened apple juice

50g (2oz) chilled butter, diced

squeeze of lemon juice

ground black pepper

steamed cabbage or kale and
mashed sweet potatoes to serve

1 Put the pork steaks on a board. Lay a slice of Parma ham or pancetta and a sage leaf on each pork steak, then secure to the meat with a wooden cocktail stick. Season with pepper.

2 Heat the oil in a large heavy-based frying pan and fry the pork for about 3–4 minutes on each side until golden brown.

3 Pour in the apple juice, stirring and scraping up the sediment from the base of the pan. Let the liquid bubble until reduced by half. Lift the pork out on to a warmed plate.

4 Return the pan to the heat, add the butter and swirl until melted into the pan juices. Add lemon juice to taste and pour over the pork. Serve with curly kale or cabbage and sweet potatoes.

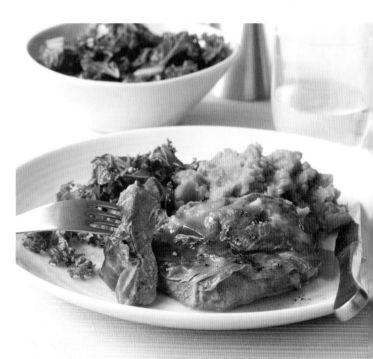

EASY		NUTRITIONAL INFORMATION		Serves
Preparation Time 5 minutes	**Cooking Time** 10 minutes	**Per Serving** 328 calories, 20g fat, (of which 9g saturates), 4g carbohydrate, 0.8g salt	Gluten free	**4**

Orange and Herb Chicken

125ml (4fl oz) orange juice

zest of 1 unwaxed orange

2 tbsp freshly chopped tarragon

2 tbsp freshly chopped flat-leafed parsley

1 tbsp olive oil

1 garlic clove, crushed

4 skinless chicken breasts

4 small orange wedges

salt and ground black pepper

brown rice and watercress to serve

1 Preheat the oven to 200°C (180°C fan oven) mark 6. In a large bowl, whisk together the orange juice, orange zest, herbs, oil and garlic. Season to taste.

2 Slash the chicken breasts several times and put in an ovenproof dish. Pour the marinade over them and top each with an orange wedge.

3 Cook in the oven for 20–30 minutes or until cooked through. Serve with brown rice and watercress.

▶ **Lemon Hummus with Black Olives**
(see page 66)
▲ **Orange and Herb Chicken**
▶ **Apple and Cranberry Strudel**
(see page 120)

Serves	EASY		NUTRITIONAL INFORMATION	
4	Preparation Time 10 minutes	Cooking Time 20–30 minutes	Per Serving 180 calories, 4g fat (of which 1g saturates), 5g carbohydrate, 0.2g salt	Gluten free Dairy free

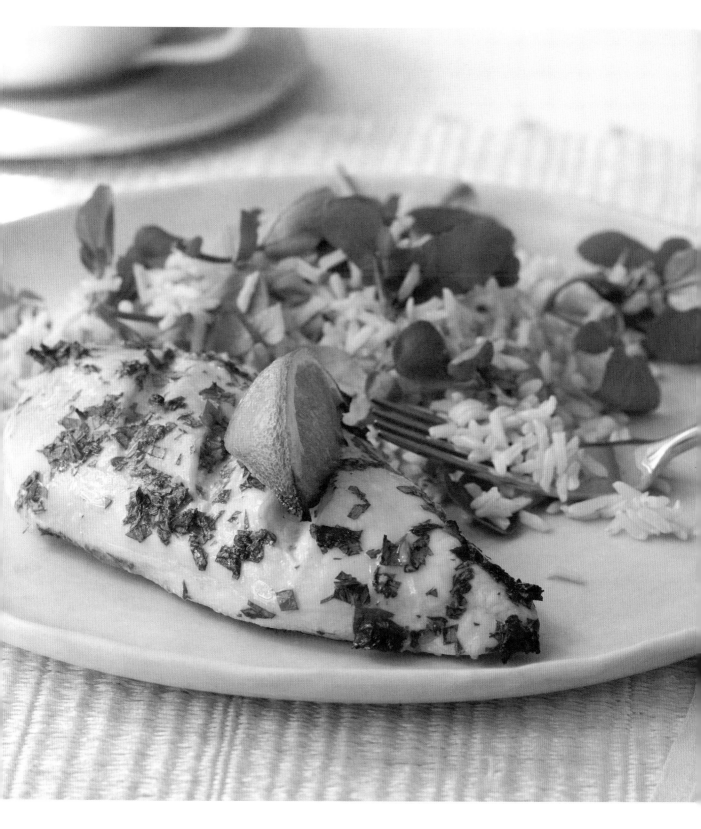

Steak with Onions and Tagliatelle

225g (8oz) tagliatelle

2 x 200g (7oz) sirloin steaks

2 red onions, thinly sliced

200g (7oz) low-fat crème fraîche

2 tbsp freshly chopped flat-leafed parsley

salt and ground black pepper

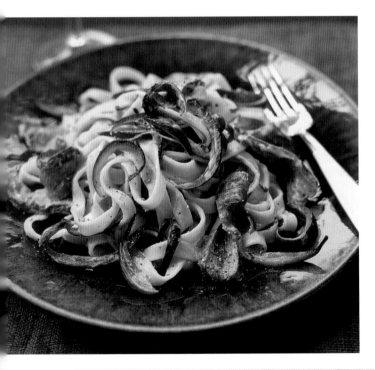

1 Cook the pasta in a large pan of boiling water according to the packet instructions; do not overcook – it should be al dente. Drain well.

2 Meanwhile, season the steaks on both sides with salt and pepper. Heat a non-stick frying pan until really hot and fry the steaks for 2–3 minutes on each side until brown but still pink inside. Remove from the pan and set aside.

3 Add the onions to the pan and stir-fry for 8–10 minutes until softened and golden. Add a little water if they're sticking. Season, reduce the heat and stir in the crème fraîche.

4 Cut the fat off the steaks and discard, then cut the meat into thin strips. Add to the pan and cook briskly for 1–2 minutes, then stir in the pasta. Add the parsley, toss again and serve immediately.

Serves 4	EASY		NUTRITIONAL INFORMATION
	Preparation Time 10 minutes	**Cooking Time** 20 minutes	**Per Serving** 557 calories, 26g fat (of which 16g saturates), 51g carbohydrate, 0.2g salt

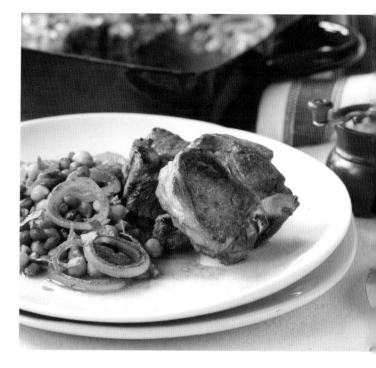

Spiced Lamb with Lentils

1 tbsp sunflower oil
8 lamb chops, trimmed of all fat
2 onions, sliced
1 tsp each paprika and ground cinnamon
400g can lentils, drained
400g can chickpeas, drained and rinsed
300ml (½ pint) lamb or chicken stock
salt and ground black pepper

1 Preheat the oven to 180°C (160°C fan oven) mark 4. Heat the oil in a large non-stick frying pan, add the chops and brown on both sides. Remove from the pan with a slotted spoon.

2 Add the onions, paprika and cinnamon and fry for 2–3 minutes. Stir in the lentils and chickpeas and season, then spoon into a shallow 2 litre (3½ pint) ovenproof dish.

3 Put the chops on top of the onion and lentil mixture and pour the stock over them.

4 Cover the dish tightly and cook in the oven for 1½ hours or until the chops are tender. Uncover and cook for 30 minutes or until lightly browned.

EASY		NUTRITIONAL INFORMATION		Serves
Preparation Time 10 minutes	Cooking Time 2 hours	Per Serving 459 calories, 17g fat (of which 6g saturates), 36g carbohydrate, 1.1g salt	Gluten free Dairy free	4

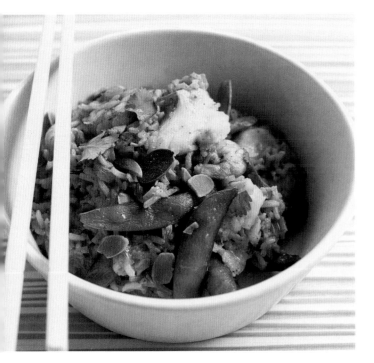

Try Something Different

There are plenty of alternatives to cod: try coley (saithe), sea bass or pollack.

Coconut Fish Pilau

2 tsp olive oil

1 shallot, chopped

1 tbsp green Thai curry paste

225g (8oz) brown basmati rice

600ml (1 pint) hot fish or vegetable stock

150ml (¼ pint) reduced-fat coconut milk

350g (12oz) skinless cod fillet, cut into bite-sized pieces

350g (12oz) sugarsnap peas

125g (4oz) cooked and peeled prawns

25g (1oz) flaked almonds, toasted

squeeze of lemon juice

2 tbsp freshly chopped coriander

salt and ground black pepper

1 Heat the oil in a frying pan, add the shallot and 1 tbsp water and fry for 4–5 minutes until golden. Stir in the curry paste and cook for 1–2 minutes.

2 Add the rice, stock and coconut milk. Bring to the boil, then cover and simmer for 15–20 minutes until all the liquid has been absorbed.

3 Add the cod and cook for 3–5 minutes. Add the sugarsnap peas, prawns, almonds and lemon juice and stir over the heat for 3–4 minutes until heated through. Check the seasoning and serve immediately, garnished with coriander.

Serves 4	EASY		NUTRITIONAL INFORMATION	
	Preparation Time 15 minutes	**Cooking Time** 30 minutes	**Per Serving** 398 calories, 7g fat (of which 1g saturates), 53g carbohydrate, 0.4g salt	Gluten free Dairy free

Cook's Tip

Serve with cherry tomatoes, grilled for 5–10 minutes until just soft, and bulgur wheat, cooked according to the packet instructions, with 2 tbsp freshly chopped parsley stirred through before serving.

Spicy Swordfish

2 red chillies, seeded and finely chopped (see page 71)

2 tbsp freshly chopped mint or coriander

3 tbsp sherry vinegar

1 tbsp olive oil

4 x 125g (4oz) swordfish steaks

8 spring onions, halved lengthways

lime wedges to serve

1 In a large, shallow dish, mix together the chillies, mint or coriander, sherry vinegar and oil. Add the swordfish steaks and coat in the dressing.

2 Preheat a griddle pan. Remove the fish from the dressing and cook, in batches, for about 4–5 minutes on each side. Transfer to plates. Add the spring onions to the griddle pan with the remaining dressing and cook for 2–3 minutes. Top the fish with the spring onions, drizzle with the juices and serve with lime wedges to squeeze over the fish.

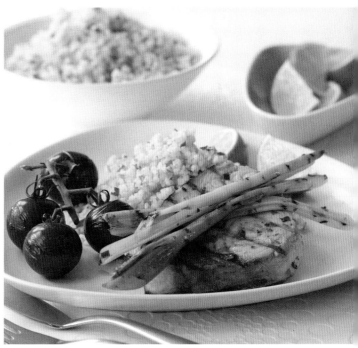

EASY		NUTRITIONAL INFORMATION		Serves
Preparation Time 15 minutes	**Cooking Time** 15–20 minutes	**Per Serving** 168 calories, 8g fat (of which 2g saturates), 1g carbohydrate, 0.4g salt	Gluten free Dairy free	**4**

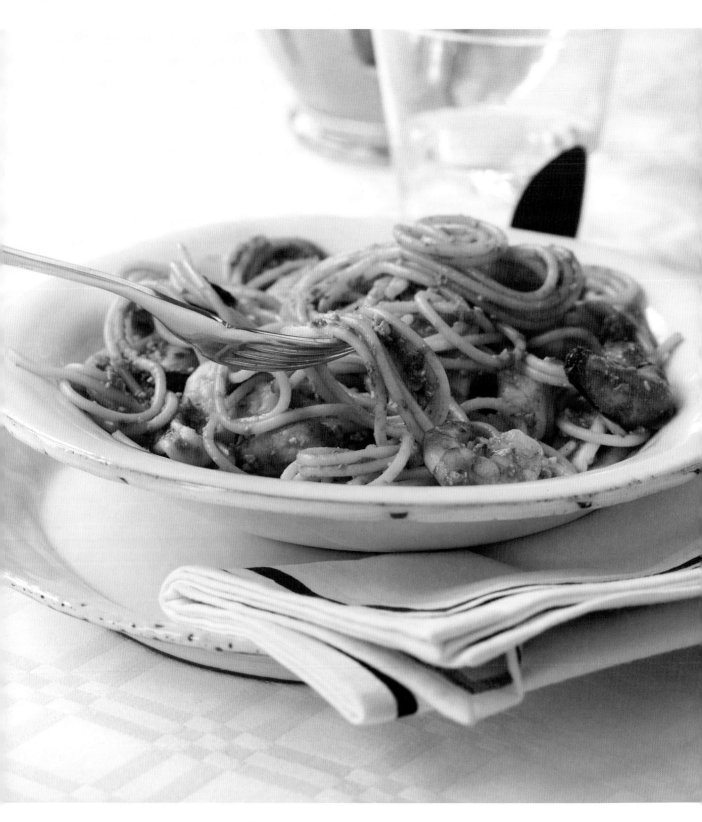

Seafood Spaghetti with Pepper and Almond Sauce

1 small red pepper

1 red chilli (see page 71)

50g (2oz) blanched almonds

2–3 garlic cloves, chopped

2 tbsp red wine vinegar

350ml (12fl oz) tomato juice

small handful of flat-leafed parsley

300g (11oz) spaghetti

450g (1lb) mixed cooked seafood, such as prawns, mussels and squid

salt and ground black pepper

1 Preheat the grill. Put the pepper and chilli under the grill and cook, turning occasionally, until the skins char and blacken. Cover and leave to cool slightly, then peel off the skins. Halve, discard the seeds, then put the flesh into a food processor.

2 Toast the almonds under the grill until golden. Add the toasted almonds and garlic to the processor with the red wine vinegar, tomato juice and half the parsley, then season with salt and pepper. Blend until almost smooth, then transfer to a large pan.

3 Meanwhile, cook the spaghetti in a pan of boiling water according to the packet instructions; keep it al dente. Heat the sauce gently until it simmers, then add the seafood. Simmer for 3–4 minutes or until the sauce and seafood have heated through, stirring frequently. Roughly chop the remaining parsley. Drain the pasta, return to the pan, then add the sauce together with the parsley and toss well.

EASY		NUTRITIONAL INFORMATION		Serves
Preparation Time 20 minutes	**Cooking Time** 25 minutes	**Per Serving** 426 calories, 9g fat (of which 1g saturates), 62g carbohydrate, 0.9g salt	Dairy free	**4**

Try Something Different

Use a different cheese, such as Stilton.

200g (7oz) baby leeks, chopped

4 spring onions, chopped

125g (4oz) baby leaf spinach

6 large eggs

4 tbsp milk

freshly grated nutmeg

125g (4oz) soft goat's cheese, chopped

1 tbsp olive oil

salt and ground black pepper

mixed salad leaves to serve

Spinach and Goat's Cheese Frittata

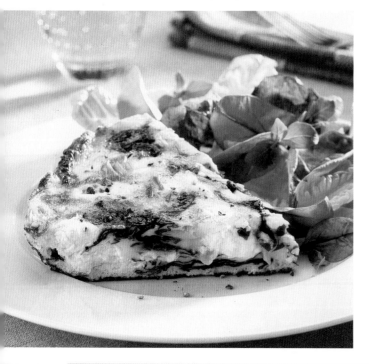

1 Preheat the grill to high. Blanch the leeks in a pan of salted boiling water for 2 minutes. Add the spring onions and spinach just before the end. Drain, rinse in cold water and dry on kitchen paper.

2 In a bowl, whisk together the eggs, milk and nutmeg. Season with salt and pepper. Stir the goat's cheese into the egg mixture with the leeks, spinach and spring onions.

3 Heat the oil in a non-stick frying pan. Pour in the frittata mixture and fry gently for 4–5 minutes, then finish under the hot grill for 4–5 minutes until the top is golden and just firm. Serve with mixed salad leaves.

Serves 4	EASY		NUTRITIONAL INFORMATION	
	Preparation Time 20 minutes	**Cooking Time** 12 minutes	**Per Serving** 280 calories, 21g fat (of which 9g saturates), 3g carbohydrate, 0.9g salt	Vegetarian Gluten free

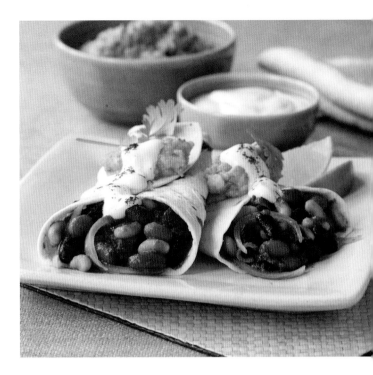

Spicy Bean and Tomato Fajitas

2 tbsp sunflower oil

1 onion, sliced

2 garlic cloves, crushed

$1/2$ tsp hot chilli powder, plus extra to garnish

1 tsp each ground coriander and ground cumin

1 tbsp tomato purée

400g can chopped tomatoes

200g can red kidney beans, drained and rinsed

400g can borlotti beans, drained and rinsed

400g can flageolet beans, drained and rinsed

150ml ($1/4$ pint) hot vegetable stock

2 ripe avocados, peeled and chopped

juice of $1/2$ lime

1 tbsp chopped coriander, plus sprigs to garnish

6 ready-made flour tortillas

150ml ($1/4$ pint) soured cream

salt and ground black pepper

lime wedges to serve

1 Heat the oil in a large pan, add the onion and cook gently for 5 minutes. Add the garlic and spices and cook for a further 2 minutes.

2 Add the tomato purée and cook for 1 minute, then add the tomatoes, beans and hot stock. Season well with salt and pepper, bring to the boil and simmer for 15 minutes, stirring occasionally.

3 Put the avocado into a bowl, add the lime juice and the chopped coriander and mash. Season to taste.

4 Warm the tortillas: either wrap them in foil and heat in the oven at 180°C (160°C fan oven) mark 4 for 10 minutes, or put on to a plate and microwave on full power for 45 seconds.

5 Spoon the beans down the centre of each tortilla. Fold up the bottom to keep the filling inside, then wrap the sides in so they overlap. Spoon on the avocado and soured cream. Sprinkle with chilli powder and coriander and serve with lime wedges.

EASY		NUTRITIONAL INFORMATION		Serves
Preparation Time 15 minutes	**Cooking Time** 25 minutes	**Per Serving** 512 calories, 20g fat (of which 6g saturates), 71g carbohydrate, 1.5g salt	Vegetarian	**6**

Baked Tomatoes and Fennel

900g (2lb) fennel, trimmed and
cut into quarters
75ml (2½fl oz) white wine
5 thyme sprigs
75ml (2½fl oz) olive oil
900g (2lb) ripe beef or plum tomatoes

1 Preheat the oven to 200°C (180°C fan oven) mark 6.
Put the fennel in a roasting tin and pour the white
wine over it. Snip the thyme sprigs over the fennel,
drizzle with the oil and roast for 45 minutes.

2 Halve the tomatoes, add to the roasting tin and
continue to roast for 30 minutes or until tender,
basting with the juices halfway through.

Cook's Tip

This is an ideal accompaniment to grilled fish or meat,
or a vegetarian frittata.

Serves 6	EASY		NUTRITIONAL INFORMATION	
	Preparation Time 10 minutes	**Cooking Time** 1¼ hours	**Per Serving** 127 calories, 9g fat (of which 1g saturates), 7g carbohydrate, 0.1g salt	Vegetarian Gluten free • Dairy free

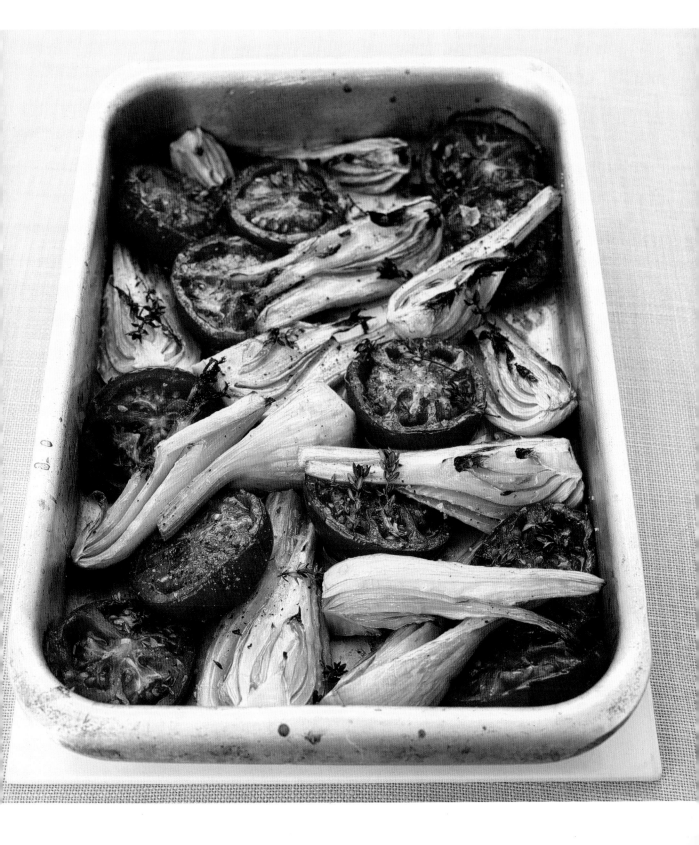

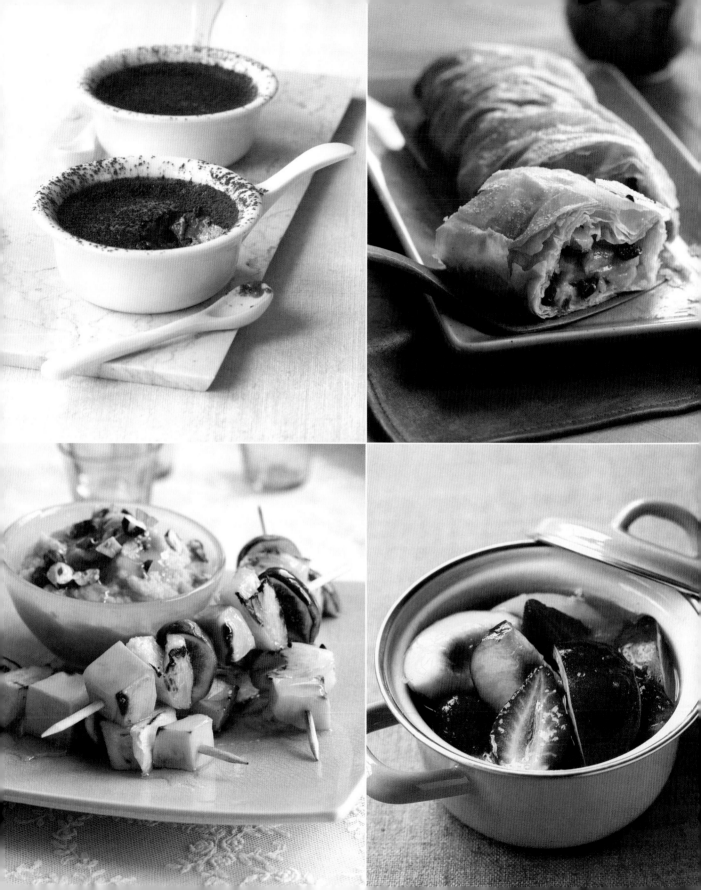

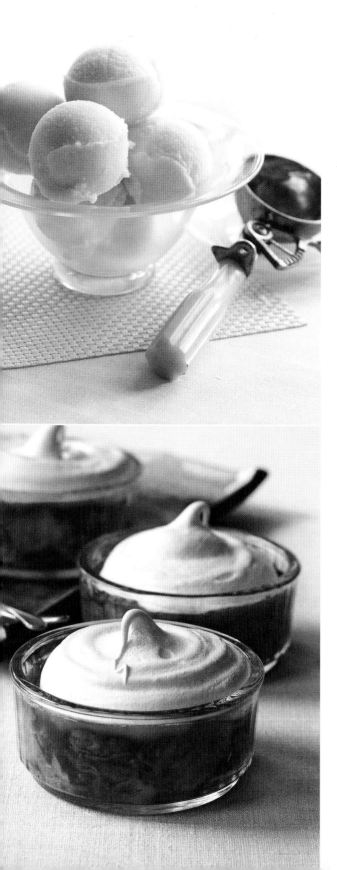

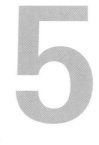

Treats

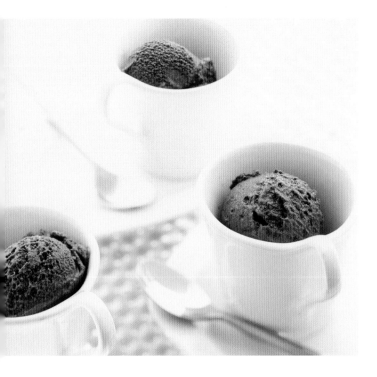

Chocolate Cinnamon Sorbet

200g (7oz) golden granulated sugar

50g (2oz) unsweetened cocoa powder

1 tsp instant espresso coffee powder

1 cinnamon stick

8 tsp crème de cacao (chocolate liqueur) to serve (optional)

1 Put the sugar, cocoa powder, coffee and cinnamon stick into a large pan with 600ml (1 pint) water. Bring to the boil, stirring until the sugar has completely dissolved. Boil for 5 minutes, then remove from the heat. Leave to cool. Remove the cinnamon stick, then chill.

2 If you have an ice-cream maker, put the mixture into it and churn for about 30 minutes until firm. Otherwise, pour into a freezerproof container and put in the coldest part of the freezer until firmly frozen, then transfer the frozen mixture to a blender or food processor and blend until smooth. Quickly put the mixture back in the container and return it to the freezer for at least 1 hour.

3 To serve, scoop the sorbet into individual cups and, if you like, drizzle 1 tsp chocolate liqueur over each portion. Serve immediately.

Serves 8	EASY		NUTRITIONAL INFORMATION	
	Preparation Time 5 minutes, plus chilling and freezing	**Cooking Time** 15 minutes	**Per Serving** 118 calories, 1g fat (of which 1g saturates), 27g carbohydrate, 0.2g salt	Vegetarian Gluten free • Dairy free

Try Something Different

Orange sorbet: replace two of the lemons with oranges.
Lime sorbet: replace two of the lemons with four limes.

Lemon Sorbet

3 juicy unwaxed lemons

125g (4oz) golden caster sugar

1 large egg white

1 Finely pare the lemon zest, using a zester, then squeeze the juice. Put the zest into a pan with the sugar and 350ml (12fl oz) water and heat gently until the sugar has dissolved. Increase the heat and boil for 10 minutes. Leave to cool.

2 Stir the lemon juice into the cooled sugar syrup. Cover and chill in the fridge for 30 minutes.

3 Strain the syrup through a fine sieve into a bowl. In another bowl, beat the egg white until just frothy, then whisk into the lemon mixture.

4 For best results, freeze in an ice-cream maker. Otherwise, pour into a shallow freezerproof container and freeze until almost frozen; mash well with a fork and freeze until solid. Transfer the sorbet to the fridge 30 minutes before serving to soften slightly.

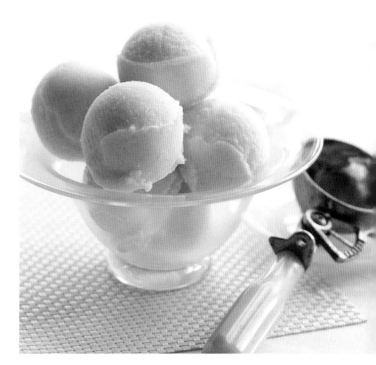

EASY		NUTRITIONAL INFORMATION		Serves
Preparation Time 10 minutes, plus chilling and freezing	**Cooking Time** 20 minutes	**Per Serving** 130 calories, 0g fat, 33g carbohydrate, 0g salt	Vegetarian Gluten free • Dairy free	4

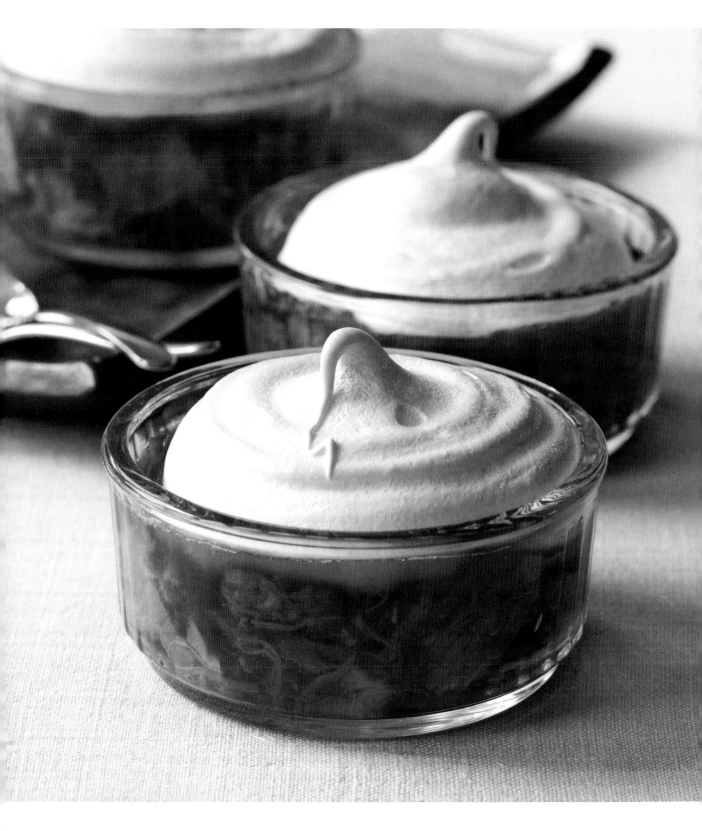

Rhubarb and Raspberry Meringue

450g (1lb) rhubarb, cut into 2.5cm (1in) pieces
75g (3oz) caster sugar
2.5cm (1in) piece stem ginger (optional), finely chopped
finely grated zest and juice of 1 orange
75g (3oz) frozen raspberries
1 large egg white

1 Place the rhubarb in a large saucepan with 25g (1oz) caster sugar, the chopped stem ginger, if using, and the orange zest. Cover and cook gently for 2–3 minutes, adding a little orange juice if necessary.

2 Add the raspberries. Spoon the mixture into four 150ml (5fl oz) ramekins or ovenproof teacups. Preheat the oven to 180°C (160°C fan) mark 4.

3 Whisk the egg white and remaining sugar together until foamy. Place the bowl over a saucepan of simmering water and continue to whisk for 5 minutes or until stiff and shiny.

4 Place a spoonful of meringue mixture on top of each ramekin and bake in the oven for 5-10 minutes or until lightly golden.

A LITTLE EFFORT

Preparation Time	**Cooking Time**
15 minutes	15–20 minutes

NUTRITIONAL INFORMATION

Per Serving
94 calories, trace fat,
22g carbohydrate, 0.1g salt

Vegetarian
Gluten free • Dairy free

Serves
4

Fruit Kebabs with Spiced Pear Dip

3 large fresh figs, quartered

1 large ripe mango, peeled, stoned and cubed

1 baby pineapple or 2 thick slices of pineapple, peeled, cored and cubed

1 tbsp dark runny honey

For the spiced pear dip

150g (5oz) ready-to-eat dried pears, soaked in hot water for about 30 minutes

juice of 1 orange

1 tsp finely chopped fresh root ginger

$\frac{1}{2}$ tsp vanilla extract

50g (2oz) very low-fat natural yogurt

$\frac{1}{2}$ tsp ground cinnamon, plus extra to dust

1 tsp dark runny honey

25g (1oz) hazelnuts, toasted and roughly chopped

1 To make the dip, drain the pears and place in a food processor or blender with the orange juice, ginger, vanilla extract, yogurt, cinnamon and 50ml (2fl oz) water and process until smooth. Spoon the dip into a bowl. Drizzle with the honey, sprinkle with the toasted hazelnuts and dust with a little ground cinnamon. Cover and set aside in a cool place until ready to serve.

2 Preheat the grill to its highest setting. To make the kebabs, thread pieces of fruit on to six 20cm (8in) wooden skewers, using at least two pieces of each type of fruit per skewer. Place the skewers on a foil-covered tray and cover the ends of the skewer with strips of foil to prevent them burning. Drizzle with honey and grill for about 4 minutes on each side, close to the heat, until lightly charred. Serve warm or at room temperature with the dip.

Serves 6	EASY		NUTRITIONAL INFORMATION	
	Preparation Time 5 minutes	**Cooking Time** 20 minutes	**Per Serving** 130 calories, 3g fat (of which trace saturates), 25g carbohydrate, 0g salt	Vegetarian Gluten free

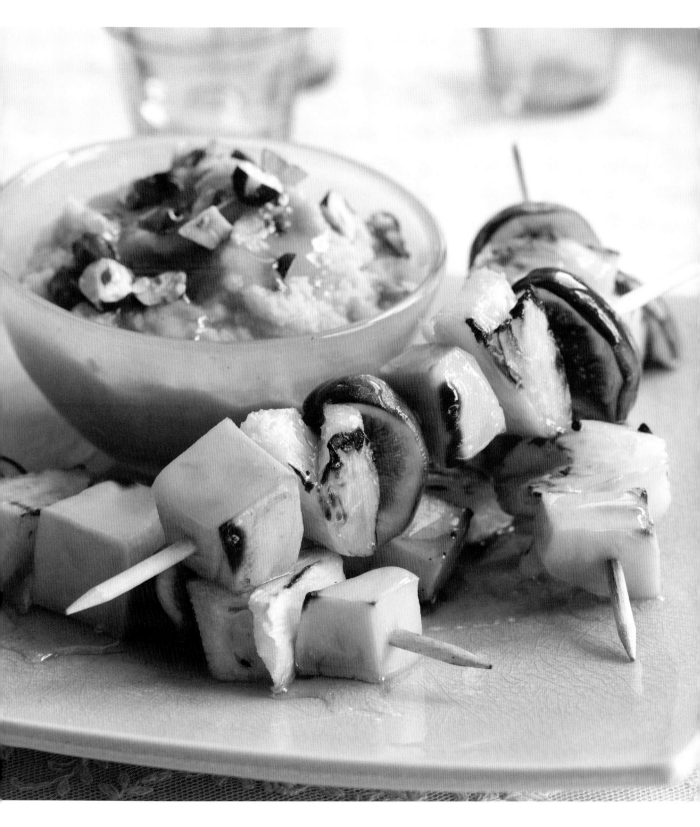

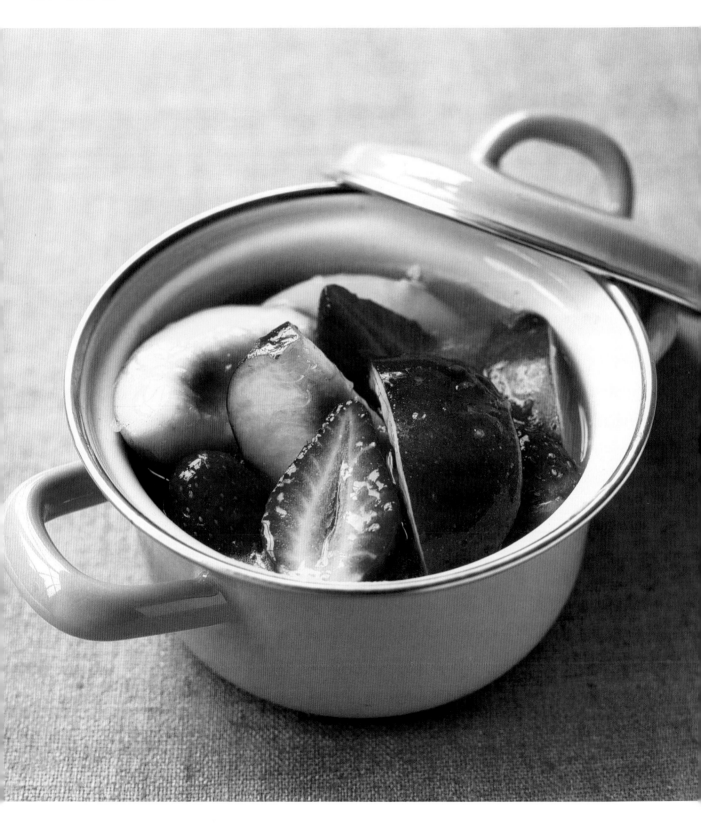

Poached Peaches and Strawberries

4 ripe peaches, halved, stoned and quartered

250ml (9fl oz) orange juice

$^1/_2$ tbsp golden caster sugar

small pinch of ground cinnamon

225g (8oz) strawberries, halved

1 Put the peaches in a pan with the orange juice, sugar and cinnamon. Simmer gently for 5 minutes. Remove the peaches with a slotted spoon and put in a bowl.

2 Let the juice bubble until reduced by half. Pour over the peaches, then cool, cover and chill. Remove from the fridge about 2 hours before serving and stir in the halved strawberries.

Try Something Different

Use nectarines instead of peaches and whole raspberries instead of the strawberries.

EASY		NUTRITIONAL INFORMATION		Serves
Preparation Time 15 minutes, plus 2 hours chilling	**Cooking Time** 10 minutes, plus cooling	**Per Serving** 78 calories, trace fat, 18g carbohydrate, 0g salt	Vegetarian Gluten free • Dairy free	**4**

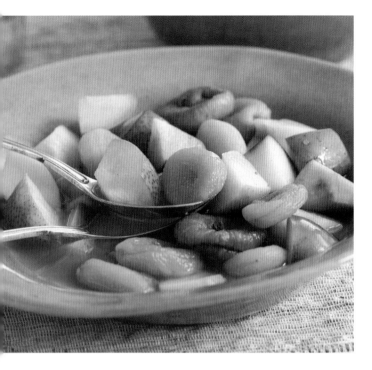

Try Something Different

Ready-to-eat prunes or 100g (3¹/₂oz) dried cranberries may be substituted for the figs.

Hot Spiced Fruit Salad

3 apples, cored and chopped

3 pears, cored and chopped

12 each ready-to-eat dried apricots and figs

juice of 2 large oranges

150ml (¹/₄ pint) apple juice

a pinch of ground cinnamon

1 star anise

1 Preheat the oven to 180°C (160°C fan oven) mark 4. Put the apples and pears into a roasting tin with the apricots and figs, the orange juice, apple juice, ground cinnamon and star anise. Stir, cover with foil and bake in the oven for 1 hour.

2 Remove the foil and bake for a further 30 minutes. Discard the star anise.

Serves 6	EASY		NUTRITIONAL INFORMATION	
	Preparation Time 10 minutes	**Cooking Time** 1½ hours	**Per Serving** 185 calories, 1g fat (0g saturates), 44g carbohydrate, 0.1g salt	Vegetarian Gluten free • Dairy free

Roasted Apples with Oats and Blueberries

4 Bramley apples

25g (1oz) pecan nuts, chopped

25g (1oz) rolled oats

50g (2oz) blueberries

2 tbsp light muscovado sugar

4 tbsp orange juice

1 Preheat the oven to 200°C (180°C fan oven) mark 6. Core the apples, then use a sharp knife to score around the middle of each (this will stop the apple from collapsing). Put the apples in a roasting tin.

2 Put the pecan nuts in a bowl together with the oats, blueberries and sugar. Mix together, then spoon into the apples, pour 1 tbsp orange juice over each apple and bake in the oven for 30–40 minutes until the apples are soft.

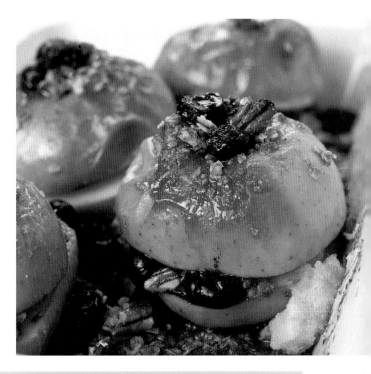

EASY		NUTRITIONAL INFORMATION		Serves
Preparation Time 15 minutes	**Cooking Time** 30–40 minutes	**Per Serving** 164 calories, 5g fat (of which trace saturates), 29g carbohydrate, 0g salt	Vegetarian Dairy free	**4**

Apple and Cranberry Strudel

700g (1½lb) red apples, quartered,
cored and thickly sliced

1 tbsp lemon juice

2 tbsp golden caster sugar

100g (3½oz) dried cranberries

6 sheets of filo pastry

1 tbsp olive oil

crème fraîche or Greek yogurt to serve

1 Preheat the oven to 190°C (170°C fan oven) mark 5. Put the apples in a bowl and mix with the lemon juice, 1 tbsp sugar and the cranberries.

2 Lay three sheets of filo pastry side by side, overlapping the long edges. Brush with a little oil. Cover with three more sheets of filo and brush again. Tip the apple mixture on to the pastry, leaving a 2cm (¾in) border all round. Brush the border with a little water, then roll up the strudel from a long edge. Put on to a non-stick baking sheet, brush with the remaining oil and sprinkle with the remaining sugar.

3 Bake in the oven for 40 minutes or until the pastry is golden and the apples are soft. Serve with crème fraîche or Greek yogurt.

Serves	EASY		NUTRITIONAL INFORMATION	
6	Preparation Time 20 minutes	Cooking Time 40 minutes	Per Serving 178 calories, 2g fat (of which trace saturates), 40g carbohydrate, 0g salt	Vegetarian Dairy free

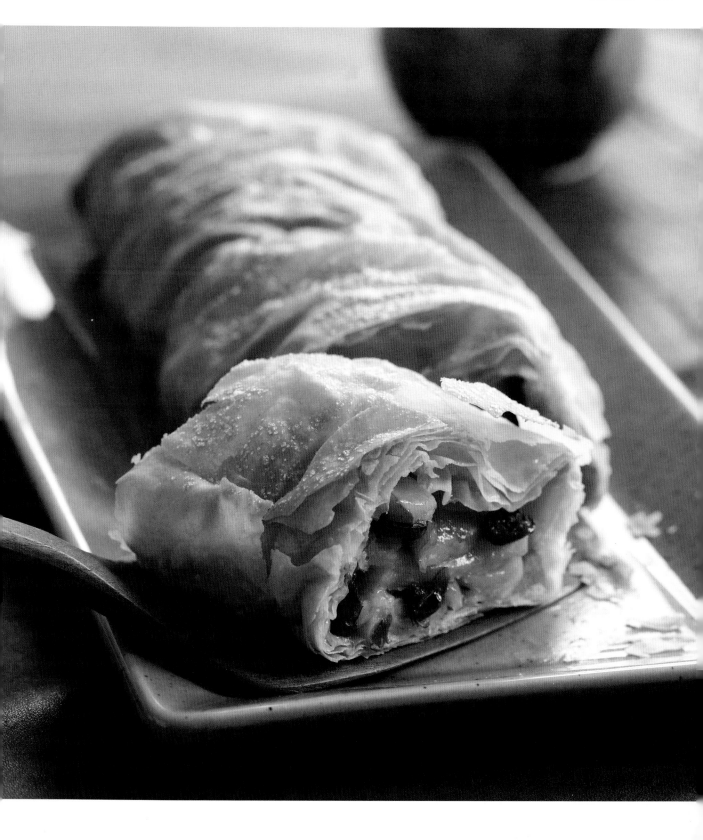

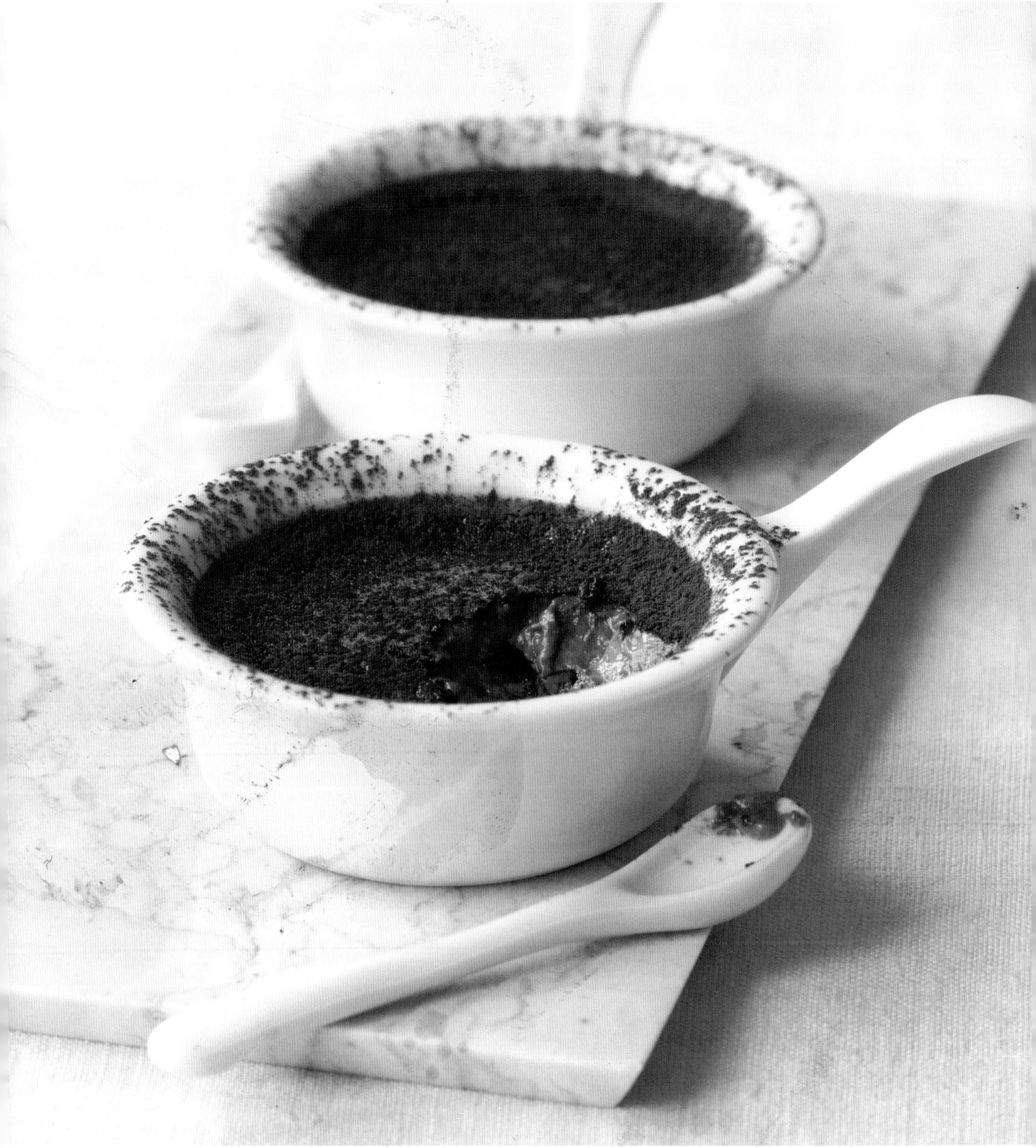

Chocolate and Prune Pudding

600ml (1 pint) skimmed milk

50g (2oz) plain chocolate, broken into tiny pieces, or chocolate chips

2 large eggs

2 large egg yolks

40g (1½oz) light brown sugar

½ tsp cornflour

2 tbsp unsweetened cocoa powder, plus extra to dust

100g (3½oz) ready-to-eat prunes, chopped

1 Preheat the oven to 170°C (150°C fan oven) mark 3. Heat the milk to simmering point, then remove from the heat. Add the broken chocolate and stir until it has melted completely.

2 In a heatproof bowl, whisk together the eggs, egg yolks, sugar, cornflour and cocoa until smooth. Gradually pour in the hot chocolate milk, stirring until it is combined.

3 Put the prunes into the base of a serving dish or individual dishes, then strain in the milk mixture through a sieve. Put the dish(es) in a roasting tin and fill the tin with boiling water so it comes halfway up the sides of the dish(es). Bake in the oven for about 30–40 minutes until just set.

4 Remove the dish(es) from the roasting tin and serve warm. Alternatively, leave to cool, then chill until ready to serve. Dust with cocoa before serving.

EASY		NUTRITIONAL INFORMATION		Serves
Preparation Time 10 minutes	**Cooking Time** 30–40 minutes	**Per Serving** 195 calories, 8g fat (of which 4g saturates), 24g carbohydrate, 0.3g salt	Vegetarian Gluten free	**6**

Try Something Different

Fresh apricots or greengages, halved and stoned, may be substituted for the cherries.

350g (12oz) stoned cherries

3 tbsp kirsch

100g (3½oz) caster sugar, plus 1 tbsp and extra to dust

4 large eggs

25g (1oz) flour

150ml (¼ pint) milk

150ml (¼ pint) single cream

1 tsp vanilla extract

butter to grease

icing sugar to dust

double cream to serve

Clafoutis

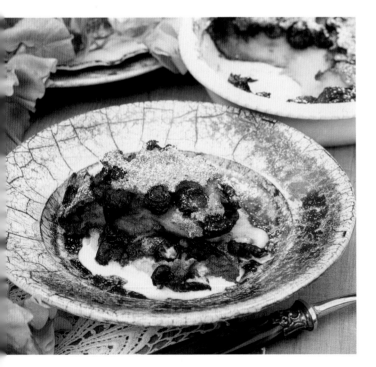

1 Put the cherries in a bowl with the kirsch and 1 tbsp sugar. Mix together, cover and set aside for 1 hour.

2 Meanwhile, whisk the eggs with the remaining caster sugar and the flour. Bring the milk and cream to the boil and pour on to the egg mixture; whisk until combined. Add the vanilla extract and strain into a bowl, cover and set aside for 30 minutes.

3 Preheat the oven to 180°C (160°C fan oven) mark 4. Lightly butter a 1.7 litre (3 pint) shallow ovenproof dish and dust with caster sugar. Spoon the cherries into the dish, whisk the batter and pour it over them. Bake in the oven for 50–60 minutes or until golden and just set. Dust with icing sugar and serve warm with cream.

Serves 6	EASY		NUTRITIONAL INFORMATION	
	Preparation Time 25 minutes, plus resting	Cooking Time 1 hour	Per Serving 235 calories, 9g fat (of which 4g saturates), 32g carbohydrate, 0.2g salt	Vegetarian

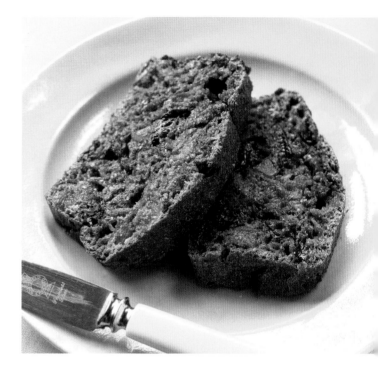

Ginger and Fruit Teabread

125g (4oz) each dried apricots, apples and
stoned prunes, chopped
300ml (½ pint) strong fruit tea
a little butter to grease
25g (1oz) stem ginger in syrup, chopped
225g (8oz) wholemeal flour
2 tsp baking powder
125g (4oz) dark muscovado sugar
1 egg, beaten

1 Put the dried fruit in a large bowl. Add the tea and
leave to soak for 2 hours.

2 Preheat the oven to 180°C (160°C fan oven) mark 4.
Grease and line the base of a 900g (2lb) loaf tin.

3 Add the remaining ingredients to the soaked fruit and
mix thoroughly. Spoon into the prepared tin and
brush with 2 tbsp cold water. Bake in the oven for
1 hour until cooked through.

4 Cool in the tin for 10–15 minutes, then turn out on
to a wire rack to cool completely. Wrap in clingfilm
and store in an airtight container. It will keep for up
to three days.

EASY		NUTRITIONAL INFORMATION		Makes
Preparation Time 15 minutes, plus 2 hours soaking	**Cooking Time** 1 hour, plus cooling	**Per Slice** 145 calories, 1g fat (of which trace saturates), 33g carbohydrate, 0g salt	Vegetarian Dairy free	**12** slices

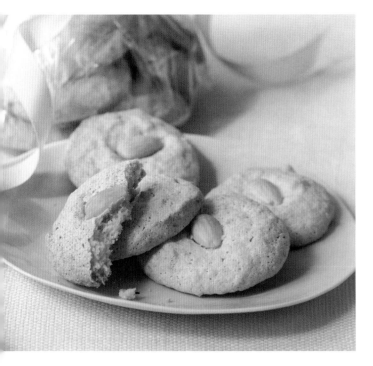

Cook's Tip

On cooling, these biscuits have a soft, chewy centre; they harden up after a few days. Once made, eat within 1 week.

Almond Macaroons

2 medium egg whites
125g (4oz) caster sugar
125g (4oz) ground almonds
¼ tsp almond extract
22 blanched almonds

1 Preheat the oven to 180°C (fan oven 160°C) mark 4 and line several baking trays with baking parchment. Whisk the egg whites until stiff peaks form. Gradually whisk in the caster sugar, a little at a time, until thick and glossy. Gently stir in the ground almonds and almond extract.

2 Spoon teaspoonfuls of the mixture on to the prepared baking trays, spacing them slightly apart. Press an almond into the centre of each one and bake in the oven for 12–15 minutes until just golden and firm to the touch.

3 Leave on the baking sheets for 10 minutes, then transfer to wire racks to cool completely. Store in airtight containers or wrap in cellophane for a gift.

Makes 22	EASY		NUTRITIONAL INFORMATION	
	Preparation Time 10 minutes	**Cooking Time** 12–15 minutes, plus cooling	**Per Macaroon** 86 calories, 6g fat (of which 1g saturates), 7g carbohydrate, 0g salt	Vegetarian Gluten free • Dairy free

Glossary

Al dente Italian term commonly used to describe food, especially pasta and vegetables, which are cooked until tender but still firm to the bite.

Baking blind Pre-baking a pastry case before filling. The pastry case is lined with greaseproof paper and weighted down with dried beans or ceramic baking beans.

Baste To spoon the juices and melted fat over meat, poultry, game or vegetables during roasting to keep them moist. The term is also used to describe spooning over a marinade.

Beat To incorporate air into an ingredient or mixture by agitating it vigorously with a spoon, fork, whisk or electric mixer. The technique is also used to soften ingredients.

Bind To mix beaten egg or other liquid into a dry mixture to hold it together.

Blanch To immerse food briefly in fast-boiling water to loosen skins, such as peaches or tomatoes, or to remove bitterness, or to destroy enzymes and preserve the colour, flavour and texture of vegetables (especially prior to freezing).

Bouquet garni Small bunch of herbs – usually a mixture of parsley stems, thyme and a bay leaf – tied in muslin and used to flavour stocks, soups and stews.

Braise To cook meat, poultry, game or vegetables slowly in a small amount of liquid in a pan or casserole with a tight-fitting lid. The food is usually first browned in oil or fat.

Caramelise To heat sugar or sugar syrup slowly until it is brown in colour; ie forms a caramel.

Chill To cool food in the fridge.

Compote Fresh or dried fruit stewed in sugar syrup. Served hot or cold.

Coulis A smooth fruit or vegetable purée, thinned if necessary to a pouring consistency.

Cream To beat together fat and sugar until the mixture is pale and fluffy, and resembles whipped cream in texture and colour. The method is used in cakes and puddings which contain a high proportion of fat and require the incorporation of a lot of air.

Croûtons Small pieces of fried or toasted bread, served with soups and salads.

Crudités Raw vegetables, usually cut into slices or sticks, typically served with a dipping sauce.

Curdle To cause sauces or creamed mixtures to separate, usually by overheating or over-beating.

Cure To preserve fish, meat or poultry by smoking, drying or salting.

Deglaze To heat stock, wine or other liquid with the cooking juices left in the pan after roasting or sautéeing, scraping and stirring vigorously to dissolve the sediment on the bottom of the pan.

Dice To cut food into small cubes.

Dredge To sprinkle food generously with flour, sugar, icing sugar etc.

Dust To sprinkle lightly with flour, cornflour, icing sugar etc.

Escalope Thin slice of meat, such as pork, veal or turkey, from the top of the leg, usually pan-fried.

Fillet Term used to describe boned breasts of birds, boned sides of fish, and the undercut of a loin of beef, lamb, pork or veal.

Flake To separate food, such as cooked fish, into natural pieces.

Folding in Method of combining a whisked or creamed mixture with other ingredients by cutting and folding so that it retains its lightness. A large metal spoon or plastic-bladed spatula is used.

Fry To cook food in hot fat or oil. There are various methods: shallow-frying in a little fat in a shallow pan; deep-frying where the food is totally immersed in oil; dry-frying in which fatty foods are cooked in a non-stick pan without extra fat; see also Stir-frying.

Garnish A decoration, usually edible, such as parsley or lemon, which is used to enhance the appearance of a savoury dish.

Gluten A protein constituent of grains, such as wheat and rye, which develops when the flour is missed with water to give the dough elasticity.

Griddle A flat, heavy, metal plate used on the hob for cooking scones or for searing savoury ingredients.

Gut To clean out the entrails from fish.

Hull To remove the stalk and calyx from soft fruits, such as strawberries.

Infuse To immerse flavourings, such as aromatic vegetables, herbs, spices and vanilla, in a liquid to impart flavour. Usually the infused liquid is brought to the boil, then left to stand for a while.

Julienne Fine 'matchstick' strips of vegetables or citrus zest, sometimes used as a garnish.

Macerate To soften and flavour raw or dried foods by soaking in a liquid, eg soaking fruit in alcohol.

Marinate To soak raw meat, poultry or game – usually in a mixture of oil, wine, vinegar and flavourings – to soften and impart flavour. The mixture, which is known as a marinade, may also be used to baste the food during cooking.

Medallion Small round piece of meat, usually beef or veal.

Mince To cut food into very fine pieces, using a mincer, food processor or knife.

Parboil To boil a vegetable or other food for part of its cooking time before finishing it by another method.

Pare To finely peel the skin or zest from vegetables or fruit.

Poach To cook food gently in liquid at simmering point; the surface should be just trembling.

Pot roast To cook meat in a covered pan with some fat and a little liquid.

Purée To pound, sieve or liquidise vegetables, fish or fruit to a smooth pulp. Purées often form the basis for soups and sauces.

Reduce To fast-boil stock or other liquid in an uncovered pan to evaporate water and concentrate the flavour.

Refresh To cool hot vegetables very quickly by plunging into ice-cold water or holding under cold running water in order to stop the cooking process and preserve the colour.

Roast To cook food by dry heat in the oven.

Roux A mixture of equal quantities of butter (or other fat) and flour cooked together to form the basis of many sauces.

Rubbing in Method of incorporating fat into flour by rubbing between the fingertips, used when a short texture is required. Used for pastry, cakes, scones and biscuits.

Salsa Piquant sauce made from chopped fresh vegetables and sometimes fruit.

Sauté To cook food in a small quantity of fat over a high heat, shaking the pan constantly – usually in a sauté pan (a frying pan with straight sides and a wide base).

Scald To pour boiling water over food to clean it, or loosen skin, eg tomatoes. Also used to describe heating milk to just below boiling point.

Score To cut parallel lines in the surface of food, such as fish (or the fat layer on meat), to improve its appearance or help it cook more quickly.

Sear To brown meat quickly in a little hot fat before grilling or roasting.

Seasoned flour Flour mixed with a little salt and pepper, used for dusting meat, fish etc., before frying.

Shred To grate cheese or slice vegetables into very fine pieces or strips.

Sieve To press food through a perforated sieve to obtain a smooth texture.

Sift To shake dry ingredients through a sieve to remove lumps.

Simmer To keep a liquid just below boiling point.

Skim To remove froth, scum or fat from the surface of stock, gravy, stews, jam etc. Use either a skimmer, a spoon or kitchen paper.

Steam To cook food in steam, usually in a steamer over rapidly boiling water.

Steep To immerse food in warm or cold liquid to soften it, and sometimes to draw out strong flavours.

Stew To cook food, such as tougher cuts of meat, in flavoured liquid which is kept at simmering point.

Stir-fry To cook small even-sized pieces of food rapidly in a little fat, tossing constantly over a high heat.

Sweat To cook chopped or sliced vegetables in a little fat without liquid in a covered pan over a low heat to soften.

Tepid The term used to describe temperature at approximately blood heat, ie 37°C (98.7°F).

Vanilla sugar Sugar in which a vanilla pod has been stored to impart its flavour.

Whipping (whisking) Beating air rapidly into a mixture either with a manual or electric whisk. Whipping usually refers to cream.

Zest The thin coloured outer layer of citrus fruit, which can be removed in fine strips with a zester.

Index